PSYCHOANALYTIC PERSPECTIVES ON SERGEI M. EISENSTEIN'S WORK

In this insightful book, Alberto Angelini shows the influence of psychoanalysis and psychology on Sergei M. Eisenstein, one of the most celebrated Russian directors, and his cinematic output.

Angelini situates Eisenstein's life and oeuvre in the history and culture of twentieth-century Russia, drawing clear parallels between his networking with key figures such as Lev Vygotsky and Aleksandr Luria. He utilises the tools of psychology with the insight of psychoanalysis to illuminate the ways in which Eisenstein understood art as an anthropological enterprise while maintaining the same dialectical philosophy as the director in highlighting the many disciplines and figures that he drew inspiration from. Angelini also looks in depth at the influence psychoanalytic theories of regression had on Eisenstein's approach to art, while examining the impact Stalinism had directly on both Eisenstein and psychoanalysis at large from the 1930s onwards.

This book is an essential resource for psychoanalysts, students, and scholars of film studies, as well as those interested in the intersection between psychoanalytic theory, cinema, and the arts.

Alberto Angelini is a psychoanalyst and psychologist based in Italy. He has worked widely in clinical practice, teaching, and supervision. Angelini graduated from and was a researcher at the National School of Cinema (CSC). He has taught Psychology at the Sapienza University of Rome and has published extensively on Russian psychoanalysis and the psychology of cinema.

PSYCHOANALYTIC PERSPECTIVES ON SERGEI M. EISENSTEIN'S WORK

Cinema and Psychoanalysis in Soviet Russia

Alberto Angelini

Translated by Barbara Antonucci

Routledge
Taylor & Francis Group
LONDON AND NEW YORK

Designed cover image: Sergei Eisenstein M. direttore russo,
Photo 12 / Alamy Foto Stock.

First published in English 2024
by Routledge
4 Park Square, Milton Park, Abingdon, Oxon OX14 4RN

and by Routledge
605 Third Avenue, New York, NY 10158

Routledge is an imprint of the Taylor & Francis Group, an informa business

Translated by Barbara Antonucci

British Library Cataloguing-in-Publication Data
A catalogue record for this book is available from the British Library

Library of Congress Cataloging-in-Publication Data
Names: Angelini, A. (Alberto), author. | Antonucci, Barbara, translator.
Title: Psychoanalytic perspectives on Sergei M. Eisenstein's work : cinema and psychoanalysis in Soviet Russia / Alberto Angelini ; translated by Barbara Antonucci.
Other titles: Sergej M. Ejzenštejn. English
Description: Abingdon, Oxon ; New York : Routledge, 2024. | Includes bibliographical references and index.
Identifiers: LCCN 2023037776 (print) | LCCN 2023037777 (ebook) | ISBN 9781032504544 (hardback) | ISBN 9781032494104 (paperback) | ISBN 9781003398554 (ebook)
Subjects: LCSH: Eisenstein, Sergei, 1898-1948—Criticism and interpretation. | Psychoanalysis and motion pictures. | Psychoanalysis in motion pictures. | Motion pictures—Psychological aspects. | LCGFT: Film criticism.
Classification: LCC PN1998.3.E34 A8513 2024 (print) | LCC PN1998.3.E34 (ebook) | DDC 791.4301/9—dc23/eng/20231023
LC record available at https://lccn.loc.gov/2023037776
LC ebook record available at https://lccn.loc.gov/2023037777

ISBN: 978-1-032-50454-4 (hbk)
ISBN: 978-1-032-49410-4 (pbk)
ISBN: 978-1-003-39855-4 (ebk)

DOI: 10.4324/9781003398554

Typeset in Times New Roman
by codeMantra

to Bianca

CONTENTS

INTRODUCTION

In the first half of the twentieth century, human science discourse was animated by a lively and hectic debate on arts and aesthetics. Sergei Mikhailovich Eisenstein was a central figure in this debate. The formal independence of cinema, within the arts, was eventually consolidated by the director's filmic and theoretical works.

The creative activity of Eisenstein – since the beginning and in a very distinctive and original manner – developed in close relation to an extensive and in-depth cognitive reflection related to the conceptual problems of arts. He confronted the theme of art and its specific thoughts, introducing new ideas. Throughout his activity, Eisenstein always cultivated a conscious and creative relationship with many theoretical and heterogeneous instances that, at his time, animated the European scene.

An extensive and general artistic and cinematographic critical perspective on Eisenstein's work is beyond the scope of the present work. Nevertheless, I believe that outlining the idea that emerges from the director's suggestion is fundamental: art represents an anthropological enterprise, structurally intrinsic to human culture, and capable of evolving throughout history. He also believed that – in its evolutionary pattern – art could be investigated by many disciplines, not only by humanities.

Because of their distinctive value in investigating multiple aspects of the human psyche, psychology and psychoanalysis represent elective instruments to support research and understanding. All this must take place, to Eisenstein's intent, following a rigorous and philosophically reliable research methodology.

This raises the *problem of method* as a fundamental presence in the Marxist philosophical heritage, embraced by Eisenstein as a hopefully resolutive tool. As a matter of fact, all over the twentieth century, epistemological issues intertwined with the very substance of scientific and humanistic disciplines. Still today, in both psychological and psychoanalytical fields – due to the many aleatory and eccentric

DOI: 10.4324/9781003398554-1

emerging ideas – the criterion of method continues to be the most important instrument to discern the validity of theoretical and clinical proposals.

Eisenstein's artistic and intellectual enterprise was wide and profound; it developed over the years and found expression, in the last part of the director's life, in a global form, as we can see in his unfinished work, whose very significant title is *Metod*. This last work, only published a few years ago, brings together different ideas and subjects studied by the director for more than a decade, from 1932 to 1948, the year of his death.

In fact, Eisenstein placed method at the basis of his theoretical enterprise from the very beginning. *Metod* was supposed to also contain his ideas on montage and directing and a study on aesthetics titled *Nonindifferent Nature*, which outlined his conceptual model and was written between 1945 and 1947. The challenging project of the director aimed to understand the meaning of each intersection between cinema and humanities as a whole.

Eisenstein was a theoretician with broad interdisciplinary interests, and in his work, he showed a tendency to intervene in areas that lie among different sciences. His deepest aspiration was to interconnect, simultaneously, anything that could make intellectual work evolve, in strict compliance with methodological criteria, drawing from anthropology and linguistics, psychology and art, aesthetics, and biology.

This superior and organic synthesis is not limited to the knowledge of each single discipline, but it dialectically occupies the territory of that speculative thought which keeps distinct opposites like reason and feeling, art and science, abstraction, and concrete action.

Cinema reassembles to recompose these crystallised oppositions, not statically, but in a dialectic and mobile form of conflict. Cinema has the *ability*, ideal and concrete, to *gain movement*.

Going even further, in Eisenstein's original intuition, "cinema discourse" is *similar* to "thinking discourse". In drawing this comparison, Eisenstein ties his ideas to the important psychological concepts of his friend Lev Vygotsky. This theoretical approach allows the cinematic instrument to entwine not only different fields of knowledge but also, and most importantly – as happens with psyche – the emotional dimension with abstract thinking.

1

THE PROBLEM OF METHOD

While some aspects related to the director's theoretical activity, such as his interest in the history of art, linguistics, and anthropology, have been broadly examined, his connection with psychology and psychoanalysis – which were emerging disciplines in the first half of the twentieth century – has been only recently considered (see Cervini, 2010).

We must remember that Eisenstein tackled the issue of a psychological approach to art in direct ways and on numerous occasions. For example, in 1940, he wrote the short essay *The Psychology of Art*, which was homonymous to an important work by Lev Vygotsky (1925a), one of the most prominent psychologists of the twentieth century and a close friend of Eisenstein. Eisenstein's essay was conceived as a list of ideas and observations aimed to elaborate a workshop project for the students of the psychologist Aleksandr Luria. Luria was a collaborator of Vygotsky's and an old friend of Eisenstein's, and he had asked the director for a specific contribution.

Even in this short essay, Eisenstein holds on to the comprehensive ideas outlined in *Metod*. He gives up a writing pattern built on a consequential and linear model to propose the vision of a "spherical book" (see Cervini, 2010, p. 16; Somaini, 2011, p. 76), which can be read starting from any single part. In this perspective, he ideally replied to Walter Benjamin, who, in *One Way Street* (1928), pointed to the possibility of creating a montage of heterogeneous and loose parts as a regulatory and non-organising hypothesis of his own book.

According to Bulgakova (2001, p. 180), the idea of a "spherical book" was inspired by the notions embedded in Gestalt psychology, particularly in Kurt Lewin's work, with whom – as we shall see –Eisenstein met. Lewin investigated the phenomena of will and action, trying to grasp their holistic sense. This was very much in tune with the director's constant idea, according to which a methodological

DOI: 10.4324/9781003398554-2

explanation, before any other sort of investigation, is at the basis of each attempt to correctly face theoretical problems. Regarding arts, Eisenstein believed that the *Fundamental Problem* (*das Grundproblem*) was related to the individuation of the laws which lie at the basis of art construction. These rules correspond, conceptually, to the laws of dialectic philosophy with their classical Hegelian legacy elaborated by Marx. This conception is all-encompassing; the same dialectical laws which regulate the activity of art also underpin the development of the individual, both from a natural and historical perspective. Human beings belong to biological nature and to historical culture, and from this, one must proceed to evaluate all the artifices that eventually assume the name of art.

From this perspective, the issue of "method" inevitably encompasses topics that cannot be limited to the artistic domain. Disciplines such as philosophy, anthropology, biology and – specially – psychology are put under scrutiny by Eisenstein in their reciprocal relations and their relation to art. Within this broad vision of human culture, we cannot differentiate, as previously done by Western tradition till the beginning of the twentieth century, art from knowledge and production activity.

Eisenstein's entire work appears as the implementation of this vision of things. According to it, artistic work is not detached from the theoretical disquisition within which different knowledge is not distinguished; dialectically, they are intimately and productively connected. In the director's perspective, the conceptual adherence to the dialectic principles corresponds – in the philosophical perspective advanced by Engels and Marx – to a recognisable practice, to the fulfilment of laws that have within them the energy and the authority of constructive axioms, in art and real life.

Eisenstein believes that making artwork has its roots in the natural world. The contents of arts, in his vision, go "from forms of existence in nature to existence as art forms". In this conception, we recognise Marx's ideas in *Economic and Philosophic Manuscripts* (1844; first published in 1932). Simultaneously, the idea of a reflection dedicated to the substantial questions of method – which needs to be distinguished from a formally structured system of knowledge – is mainly consistent with Engels' positions, which, more than Marx, highlighted the necessity to differentiate within the Hegelian philosophy, "method" from "system" of knowledge.

According to Engels, the method, more than anything, is capable of investigating nature in its single parts, taken separately. Unfortunately, though, this method does not favour a global vision; in fact, it entails

> the habit of observing natural objects and processes in isolation, apart from their connection with the vast whole; of observing them in repose, not in motion; as constants, not as essentially variables; in their death, not in their life. This way of looking at things [...] begot the narrow, metaphysical mode of thought thinking [...]. To the metaphysician, things and their mental reflexes, ideas, are isolated, are to be considered one after the other and apart from each other, are objects of investigation fixed, rigid, given once for all ... [For the metaphysician] a thing

> exists or does not exist; a thing cannot at the same time be itself and something else. Positive and negative absolutely exclude one another; cause and effect stand in a rigid antithesis one to another.
>
> *(Engels, 1878; Engl. transl., p. 22)*

Eisenstein's whole activity, as Vygotsky's work from which Eisenstein drew inspiration, is aimed to overcome this crystallised fixity and recover the value of movement and dialectics in every natural and human expression. From a methodological perspective, at the time, this could correspond to a response and reaction to the triumph of the Pavlovian conditioned reflex, which encompassed any issue related to the historical complexity of the human subject. Vygotsky had been very critical of reflexology, opposing the mechanical application of reflex theory in complex situations. In *Consciousness as a Problem for the Psychology of Behavior* (1925a), Vygotsky states:

> 'Reflex' is an abstract concept. From the methodological viewpoint it is extremely valuable, but it cannot become the fundamental concept of psychology viewed as the concrete science of human behavior [...] [Man] is not at all a skin sack filled with reflexes and *the* brain is not a hotel for conditional reflexes that happen to pass by.
>
> *(Engl. transl., 1997, p. 66)*

He also put forward some critical points in relation to psychoanalysis, even though some years before, he had sympathised with Freud's ideas and supported them. In this work, he expresses the preoccupation that psychoanalysis cannot become a "vision of the world". From a methodological perspective, the same was true for the Gestalt theory. Behind this attitude stood the idea that it was not methodologically correct to try to interpret the complexity of the historical and social world by applying, mechanically, one or another doctrine.

Vygotsky expressed these ideas in *The Historical Meaning of the Crisis in Psychology* (1927), written after a period spent in the Zakharino hospital, over 100 km from Moscow. Even Eisenstein, seeing his friend after his stay in the hospital, distanced himself from the reflexological perspective. The film director, previously sympathetic to Pavlovism as a pupil of Meyerhold, who had advocated this perspective in his training of the actor, welcomed the Engelsian vision, advocating a method capable of interpreting nature and the world as a whole.

This is the idea of dialectical materialism. To this idea belong those laws, formulated by Hegel, which concern not only the movement of thinking but also the physical world itself, in its reality, in nature, and the concrete life of humankind. If movement is the relentless engine of ideas and life in its every expression, including the artistic one, then it is comprehensible how the idea of synthesis must always be considered impermanent and never given a fixed way. This is why, according to Eisenstein, the dialectical method represents a solution for the "fundamental problem" of art, that is to say, the methodological research of laws that are at the basis of its construction. Through this method, he sees the possibility of overcoming every form of metaphysical dualism that manifests in the artistic field.

On a biographical level, the outlines of the ideas which then were to be found in *Metod* make their first appearance in 1935, the same year the director returned to his homeland after a long journey through Europe and America.

Eisenstein maintained an interest in psychoanalysis all his life, but already in the early 1930s, the name of Freud had become a taboo in the USSR. In his letters, he asked his friends abroad to send him new books on psychoanalysis (see Bulgakova, 2001, p. 172). We find traces of this interest in *Metod*, written till the director's death in 1948, leaving the legacy of an important work, though unfinished and not organic. In the same period, many important works were published, such as *Montazh* (1935–1937, henceforth *General Theory of Montage*), *Montage 38* (1938), *Vertical Montage* (1940) and *Nonindifferent Nature* (1945–1947). We must look at these works and the methodological notes outlined in *Psychology of Art* to understand the connection between his writings and *Metod* since all of them contribute to outline the director's general vision.

The adoption of a dialectical method allows Eisenstein to overcome the principle of non-contradiction, which does not allow to grasp movement, seen as characteristic of thought and, above all, material reality. These concepts are connected, philosophically and symbolically, to cinema and to the technical peculiarities which characterise it: montage. The topic of montage was always central in Eisenstein's work. He emblematically stated: "To determine the nature of montage is to solve the specific problem of cinema" (Eisenstein, 1949, p. 48).

The montage process, from the director's viewpoint, allows the art of filmmaking to confront itself for the first time and concretely, with the real reproduction of movement as a phenomenon both and simultaneously *subjective* – as a movement of thought – and *objective* – as the movement of individuals, things, and the world. The two dimensions on the screen are evoked in their mutual interpenetration. Even in this case, Eisenstein embraces the Engelsian idea of one principle which regulates forms of natural movement, history, and thought. It is a unitary vision of the world, or rather a sort of real *Weltanschauung*, although with the requirement to have scientific foundations. According to it, the process of artistic production and the whole development of man as an individual and as a species, must respond to the rules of dialectical materialism. This perspective also concerns the passage from quantity to quality, i.e., the construction of the organic artwork, defined for the continuity between inorganic (the work) and the different forms of the living. The progressive introduction of qualitatively different compositional elements produces artistic synthesis. By virtue of this complex vision, inspired by the dialectical philosophy of Marxism, Eisenstein's attention is drawn to areas not directly related to art itself, such as historical, anthropological, and psychological research.

On this concrete level, there cannot be borders among the different instances which contribute to the development of humankind. It is necessary, both in a phylogenetic and ontogenetic sense, to overcome the paradigm of a linear evolutive movement. With respect to thought, this means abandoning the privilege given to sensible logic, typically identified with metaphysics, to embrace a historical vision which involves, at the same time, man and nature. This point of view uses an alternative model, which keeps progressive and regressive movements together.

On the level of Eisenstein's theoretical interests, this corresponds to progressively getting closer to those expressions of primitive thought that he defines as "prelogical", a definition drawn from Lévy-Bruhl (1910). Similarly, he is attracted to those forms of social and cultural organisation, as in the case of Mexican peoples, still distant from the capitalistic system. To understand human history, as well as art, an elaborated theoretical model is paramount, a model which is in harmony with the philosophical idea of a double movement: on the one hand, progressive, towards higher strata of consciousness, on the other hand regressive, towards the lower layers. The elements at stake, thus, exist simultaneously, regression and progression. Conservation of past and future innovation live together. In the same way, pre-logic and rational thought live together in the making of art, seen as a means, among others, through which human society is created.

By virtue of this methodological principle, which involves, universally, all the disciplines and human history, Eisenstein's ideas and interests had no boundaries.

As aforementioned, Eisenstein took an interest in biological and anthropological questions, and his work is a demonstration that he never set conceptual boundaries, but, within the present work, the focus is on the relationship between the director, psychology, and psychoanalysis.

Eisenstein focused on psychological phenomena to define the conditions that make artwork *effective*.

He first familiarised himself with the topics of reflexological psychology introduced by Pavlov and Bekhterev that, along with other instances, flowed into "Biomechanics" based on Meyerhold's ideas. With Meyerhold, who can be considered his artistic mentor, young Eisenstein founded the theatre section of the Proletkult. This "Cultural, Educational and Proletarian Organization", strongly favoured by the Marxist theoretician Aleksandr Bogdanov, after the revolutionary victory, became dependent on "The People's Commissariat for Education". Bordwell recalls that "during 1921–22 theatre season Eisenstein studied at Meyerhold's workshop, where he learned biomechanics. Meyerhold publicly announced the technique in the spring of 1922, emphasizing the training sessions of the actor's reflexes" (Bordwell, 1993, p. 116). Eisenstein had met this great protagonist of the Russian theatrical avant-garde when he was young. In his thoughts, he summoned, besides reflexology, constructivism, the theory of emotions by William James, instances of oriental drama, and Taylor's ideas (see Somaini, 2011, p. 7). Etkind put forward the idea that Eisenstein had developed a sort of Oedipus complex towards his teacher Vsevolod Meyerhold and Sigmund Freud, and he stated, quoting the director:

> Eisenstein related how Freud had helped him understand his relation with his own teacher, Vsevolod Meyerhold. "It was an oedipal complex like the play of passions within Freud's own school. The "sons" were attacking their father more in response to his "regime of tyranny". And the father in this case was more like Saturn, who devoured his own children, than like Oedipus's harmless father … Isn't this the source of the image of the horde that eats the eldest of its kind? … The same sort of grand old man in the center, infinitely charming as a master and foully malicious as a person; the *same* discord, a rupture in initial harmony; … the same impetuous growth of individualities around him. The same intolerance for any sign of independence"
>
> *(Etkind, 1997, p. 316)*

Eisenstein wanted to work, introspectively, on his own father. Etkind suggests that Eisenstein's father failed in explaining young Serëža issues related to sexuality, while Meyerhold, afterwards, did not give him answers on the problems raised by art. Freud represented Meyerhold, and Meyerhold symbolised Eisenstein's father (Etkind, 1997, p. 316). In fact, Eisenstein's father, Mikhail Osipovich, in favour of tzarism, at the end of the civil war and with the victory of the Bolsheviks, decided to move to Germany. Young Sergej, on the eve of the October Revolution, abandoned the faculty of architecture to enlist in the Red Army.

Eisenstein, like many other intellectuals of the first half of the twentieth century, was vividly attracted by psychoanalysis. On some occasions, as we shall see further on, he even asked to undergo some therapeutic treatments with members of the psychoanalytical movement.

Paradoxically, in that period, a minor stream of psychoanalytical thought discouraged in-depth treatment of subjects with a strong artistic attitude, with the idea that it could impact negatively on the person's creativity. At the time, Etkind stated

> In the Moscow intelligentsia there is a legend that continues to circulate today (one that might *very* well be true) that a certain Moscow psychoanalyst turned Sergey Eisenstein away on the same grounds, saying that after psychoanalysis the filmmaker would have to look for an accounting job in the State Planning Committee.
>
> *(Etkind, 1997, p. 60)*

On a more general historical level, the filmmaker was certainly deeply influenced by psychoanalytical thinking but was also reached by other concepts related to psychology. For example, as previously stated, he encountered the principles of reflexology, of Soviet matrix, studies on hypnosis (Angelini, 1992, p. 53 ff., 2020, pp. 216, 228) and the ideas of Henri Bergson (Cervini, 2010, p. 97 ff.).

Meyerhold was deeply interested in reflexology and developed biomechanics, a formative method aimed to learn and investigate the art of acting based on reflexology notions. Being in contact with Meyerhold, Eisenstein showed great interest in reflexology.

The idea of the "Montage of Attraction", which will be further illustrated, originates from a physiological perspective; the "attraction" is a sensory effect that is supposed to reach the spectators.

But from 1925, with the first publication in Russian and German of Friedrich Engels' *Dialectics of Nature*, reflexology began to be polemically accused of mechanism by some Soviet theoreticians.

Eisenstein was also reached by the ideas of Gestalt psychology. Although he was initially influenced mostly by psychoanalysis, he was also very interested in the ideas circulating and related to psychology. He was attracted by anything which could enhance the effective development of the psychology of art.

Eisenstein met Wolfgang Köhler and Kurt Lewin. As will be explained later, he met both in 1930 after giving a lecture at the Institute of Psychology of the University of Berlin. Berlin, at the time, was the second most important centre of psychoanalytical research after Wien, and that is where the first actual encounter between cinema and psychoanalysis took place. In 1922, Fritz Lang made *Doctor Mabuse*, among the most notorious examples of expressionist cinema, whose protagonist is a criminal and violent psychoanalyst who ends up, luckily, trapped in his own nightmares. In 1926, Georg Wilhelm Pabst completed *Secrets of a Soul*, a film with strong psychoanalytical traits. Pabst had even asked Freud for advice, but Freud refused the offer. But Karl Abraham, at the time director of the Psychoanalytic Institute of Berlin and Hans Sachs, a close friend of Eisenstein, accepted. Sachs even wrote a booklet accompanying the film (see Eppensteimer, Fallend and Reichnayr, 1987, p. 129). In that period, Kenneth Macpherson was also in Berlin and in 1930, he directed the film *Borderline*. The film – which was thought lost but was recovered in Switzerland in 1983 – is considered an original experimental production.

In 1927, Macpherson and Winifred Bryer (pseudonym of the author Annie Winifred Ellerman) launched the magazine *Close Up*. The magazine had a strong interest in the relationship between psychoanalysis and film, and the editors published several works by Eisenstein and Sachs. Winifred Bryer was also treated by Sachs until he moved to Boston in 1932. In 1928, Sachs published a short essay titled *Psychology of the Movies* wherein, among other things, he commented on Eisenstein's *Battleship Potemkin* (1925) and Vsevolod Pudovkin's *Mother* (1926) from a psychoanalytical perspective. The article was translated into German the following year. The film *Battleship Potemkin* was drastically boycotted in Russia. Konstantin Shvedchikov, director of Sovkino, the organisation that distributed films in the USSR, was a modest party bureaucrat who knew nothing about cinema and was attracted by foreign low-quality films. In addition, he was also an anti-semite, scornfully called by Eisenstein "The nobleman of Jerusalem". For long, Shvedchikov opposed the distribution of *Battleship Potemkin*. On that occasion, even Mayakovski, a friend of the director, took the position, but the obscure bureaucrat was immovable; only after much pressure, he allowed the distribution and sent some copies to Berlin, sure of the unsuccess of the product. The Berlin premiere took place at the Apollo Theatre on the twenty-ninth of April 1926, and among the spectators there was Max Reinhardt. The success was outstanding; paradoxically, the film was even appreciated by the ministry of nazi propaganda Joseph Goebbels, although, by acknowledging its convincing power in favour of Bolshevism, in 1933, he had the film seized.

Close Up was printed in English. Eisenstein published several articles in the magazine, and in 1929, he often met Macpherson. The latter, in several articles that appeared on *Close Up* in 1930, often commented on Sachs' and Eisenstein's ideas. He claimed to have attempted, in his film *Borderline* (1930), a synthesis between Eisenstein's montage theory and Sachs' views on the psychology of audience perception (see Bulgakova, 1989, p. 81).

In 1930, the director was in Paris, where René Allendy, vice president of the French Psychoanalytic Society and professor at the Sorbonne, had organised a screening of the film *Old and New* at the university. Police prevented the screening. Allendy, Anaïs Nin's analyst and friend of Artaud at the time, was writing a book on the psychology of cinema, and Eisenstein met him on several occasions to exchange ideas.

During his stay in Berlin in 1930, the director approached Gestalt. We should not forget that Aleksandr Luria and Lev Vygotsky, his two psychologist friends, had confronted this school.

Between 1930 and 1931, Luria invited Koffka to take part in his second expedition for psychological research in the Asian Soviet Republics. In his autobiography, the Russian psychologist expressed the idea that Koffka, due to his Gestalt education, could not "grasp what was the fundamental aim of the expedition, and was unable to participate in it in a creative and active way" (Luria, 1982; Ital. transl., p. 49).[1] Vygotsky partially criticised Gestalt, but he positively valued the original aim of Gestalt, designed to contrast the vitalist and mechanistic perspectives. According to these perspectives, human beings were considered machines or metaphysical subjects. According to Vygotsky, Gestalt contributed to a theory of perception and thought based on concrete facts. However, he believed that the concept of structure, at the basis of Gestalt, could assume eternal and metaphysical characteristics. For this reason, in an overall evaluation, Vygotsky wrote that the Gestalt concepts "from the point of view of the historic pattern of science, were not capable to actually overcome mechanism and vitalism" (Vygotsky, 1932b; Ital. transl., pp. 140, 141). Later on, in 1934, the Soviet psychologist wrote the introduction to the translation in the Russian language of Kurt Koffka's *The Growth of the Mind* (1928), stating the same beliefs. He asserted that, even if Gestalt could represent progress over the mechanism of the stimulus-response theories, some of its exponents fell into the error of advocating a theory based on a single development factor and a single explicative principle. They tried to account for all levels of psychological functioning, based on the notion of *structure*, or *Gestalt*, neglecting the fundamental qualitative differences in the functioning ways manifesting in different domains of psychological phenomena.

In a more general sense, we should not forget that Vygotsky, a great theoretician of cognition, was always distinctly unrelated to the theoretical positions influenced by mechanism. In the words of Bakhurst,

> It is beyond doubt that Vygotsky admired science. The key issue, however, is what he understood by science. His writings suggest that he took scientific explanation to have three distinguishing marks (see Vygotsky, 1927, chapter fifteen, section two). Scientific explanations are (1) naturalistic in that they invoke only phenomena that are constituents of the natural world; (2) causal in that they explain events by showing how they are necessitated by prior conditions; and (3) systematic in that their intelligibility depends on a background system of theoretical knowledge. It is crucial to note, however, that Vygotsky did not take a narrow view of nature, cause, and system. His conception of causation is not mechanistic, and he was consistently hostile to reductive modes of explanation, as is evident from his dialectical conception of development through qualitative transformation. He understood well that any naturalistic monism must admit diverse forms of causal interaction and adopt relaxed, open-minded strategies to integrate the various elements in our conception of the world to reflect the unity of nature. It is also important that Vygotsky did not disparage "nonscientific" modes of understanding. He was not the kind of rationalist who preferred to see human beings as cold, abstract reasoners. On the contrary, he insisted on the importance of the emotions in guiding and informing cognition.
>
> *(Bakhurst, 2007, p. 68)*

Historically, the work of Vygotsky began to be studied and discussed again by Russian psychologists in the so-called period of the political and cultural "thaw" after Stalin's death. In Italy, the first integral translation in Italian of his fundamental work *Thinking and Speech* (1934) was published only in 1990, edited by Luciano Mecacci. And the second translation in the Western world was in German in 2002. Today, he is the most studied twentieth-century psychologist and scientific research on Vygotsky, and his work gathers a lot of scientific literature.

Great attention was given to Vygotsky's ideas on the relationship between psychology and scientific method. This great attention to the methodological premises came from Marxism and, on a conceptual level, was influenced by Engels' *Dialectics of Nature*, published posthumously in 1925, and by the ideas on method and dialectics outlined by Lenin in 1909 in *Materialism ed Empirio-Criticism*.

This attention on epistemological questions, aimed to avoid slips, even unconsciously, towards the simplifications of metaphysics and mechanism, belonged to the entire Soviet culture, both in the field of humanistic knowledge and in the field of science.

Eisenstein was also aware that any proposal founded on an uncertain methodological basis would be useless and have a negative fate. For this reason, many theoretical aspects of his thoughts are connected to Marxist dialectics and ideas coming from psychoanalysis and Soviet psychology. There are also some connections to Gestalt authors, like Lewin and Koffka (see Del Rio and Alvarez, 2007), while other approaches (see Greenfield, 1975; Bulgakova, 1989) that connect the director's idea to Gestalt appear disproportionate.

With concern to Gestalt, Eisenstein's positions recall – for the substance of his interests – the general ideas expressed by Vygotsky. To better understand these conceptual aspects and the differences between Gestalt and Eisenstein, it is useful to briefly outline the hypothesis of the most representative figure of Gestalt related to cinema: Rudolf Arnheim. He was a contemporary of Eisenstein, although they never had a head-to-head confrontation.

Arnheim, psychologist and art critic, is universally known as a defender of the expressive autonomy of cinema compared to other art forms. His research, presented mostly in *Film as Art* (1933–1938), focuses on the relation between the cinematographic perception and the psychological model by which he intends to explain its functioning. Arnheim's idea on cinematographic perception was, overall, coherent with the principles of Gestalt psychology, which he himself defined, in the introduction, as a Kantian tendency of perception studies. On the same page, he recalls having been a student of two major Gestalt theorists: Max Wertheimer and Wolfgang Köhler. Gestalt's Kantianism can be considered, from Vygotsky' and Eisenstein's perspective, the intrinsic cause of the limits of their theoretical proposals. We should not forget that, analogously, Lenin, in *Materialism and Empirio-Criticism* (1909), had fought a harsh philosophical battle against the empirio-criticist theories of Kantian derivation.

Arnheim,

> in tune with the Gestalt hypothesis which attributes to the mind its own operative ability in relation to the perceptive phenomenon, criticizes those tendencies that see cinema as a mere tool to automatically record reality, substantially conditioned by its technical nature; while in cinema in every shot, in each frame, down to the single photogram, the choices – not only technical – selected by the director determine specific perceptive and aesthetical results which are not only a recording of reality …This perspective, on a perceptive level, underlies the director's ability to process material *in* tune with the operational structures of the mind.
>
> *(Angelini, 1989, p. 51)*

While it is certainly true that cinema represents more than a mere tool of automatic recording of reality, expanding Arnheim's conceptions, the work of the director and the artist, in general, should be at the utmost *independent* from reality. The director should respect, firstly, the "operational abilities" of the mind. In fact, Arnheim did not believe that the real world had "the formal precision that in the work of art presents – by means of the sensory data – the subject and its qualities in a clear-cut, expressive way" (Arnheim, 1933; Engl. transl., p. 200). This is due to the fact that "physical reality shapes and assembles things and events only in approximation of the pure, authentic 'ideas', that are at the bottom of the empirical world" (Arnheim, 1933; Engl. transl., p. 200).

Clearly, these positions are very distant from Eisenstein's. In the years Arnheim worked and wrote, the director had already related the language of cinema to infantile and primitive expressive forms. Coherent with his Marxist philosophical ideas, he had adhered to Vygotsky's psychological ideas. Vygotsky, as we shall see, conceived and promoted the *Cultural-Historical Theory of Development:* according to it, the human mind, in its higher psychological functions, is determined by the context of concrete historical reality. From this approach, we come to understand how, for Eisenstein, the human mind as well as the director's mind – who carries on the filming and editing – cannot be alien to the historical and social context within which artwork takes shape and in which the director expresses himself. This idea has a universal value; when the director refers to dialectical philosophy, he does not speak of a dimension which belongs only to film work, but he deals with the complex relations that involve film, the author, and the social context within which the work is realised. As Eisenstein writes: "The final order is inevitably determined, consciously or unconsciously, by the social premises of the maker of the film-composition" (Eisenstein, 1949, p. 4). This is a very distant perspective compared to the Gestalt structures outlined by Arnheim, which are intrinsic to the human mind and the universe.

Eisenstein's psychological interests are focused on psychoanalysis and Vygotsky's thoughts. Both these theoretical proposals were condemned by the Soviet regime theoreticians. These ideas conceptually represented psychological and dialectical proposals that were antagonists to mechanism and metaphysics.

Note

1 In the English version of Luria's autobiography (1979), this note on Koffka is omitted.

2

PSYCHOANALYSIS IN RUSSIA

Looking at the relation between Eisenstein and psychoanalysis, we can see that – as with other great artists of the early twentieth century – psychoanalysis represented the great aspiration to organise, in a scientific or at least sensible way, problems related to the inner subjectivity of the human being. The artistic phenomenon appeared as a research field that psychoanalysis could help clarify. The fundamental problem concerned the need to guarantee a secure *methodological basis* for any theoretical proposal related to art as related to the person who makes it or receives it. The issue of method had to be faced scientifically and rationally, avoiding leaps into metaphysics or slips into gross mechanistic materialism.

Although he did not detect the connections between Eisenstein, Vygotsky and psychoanalysis, in 1980, Carroll wrote:

> Theorists like Eisenstein, Pudovkin, and Balàzs, wanted to establish a scientific program for cinema theory. Eisenstein especially attempted to integrate the scientific study of film with psychology, sociology, and linguistics. He believed that the scientific method could be applied, and indeed *had* to be applied to the study of art: science and art could not be separated from each other.
>
> *(Carrol, 1980, p. 8)*

The names of Eisenstein and Pudovkin are juxtaposed, but, as a matter of fact, despite the common reference to Marxism, the two nourished very different ideas on the art of cinema. With concern to montage criteria, for example, they had two different conceptual points of view. Eisenstein wrote:

> The earliest conscious film-makers, and our first film theoreticians, regarded montage as a means of description by placing single shots one after the other

DOI: 10.4324/9781003398554-3

> like building-blocks. The movement within these building-block shots, and the consequent length of the component pieces, was then considered as rhythm. A completely false concept! This would mean the defining of a given object solely in relation to the nature of its external course. The mechanical process of splicing would be made a principle … According to this definition, shared even by Pudovkin as a theoretician, montage is the means of *unrolling* an idea with the help of single shots: the "epic" principle. In my opinion, *however*, montage is an idea that arises from the collision of independent shots–shots even opposite to one another: the "dramatic" principle.
>
> *(Eisenstein, 1949, pp. 48, 49)*

Epic and dramatic refer to formal aspects, not to the contents or the plot. In sum, Pudovkin considered montage as an instrument to develop, *in a linear way*, an idea through cinema discourse, while Eisenstein *contentiously* calls for a cinema of confrontation and clash. In this, he seeks the cinematic expression of the psychological conflicts. Montage must be conflictual, like the individual's emotions and thoughts, coherently with the idea of conflict coming from materialistic dialectical philosophy. As he wrote in A *General Theory of Montage*, devised between 1935 and 1937: "The principle of cinema is a reproduction in terms of film, footage, framing and projection rhythm of an indispensable and profoundly original process, which characterises, in general, consciousness from its first steps in the assimilation of reality" (Eisenstein, 1985; Ital. transl., p. 144). This process makes explicit, through cinema, a *sense* which was enclosed in the director's mind. Nevertheless, for this reason, the process of montage cannot be alien to the social and historical context in which the cinematographic work is created and in which authors express themselves. Talking about montage, Eisenstein openly refers to Engel's *Dialectics of Nature*, but the dialectics to which he refers is not only intrinsic to the nature of the filmic realisation, but it concerns all the complex relations that belong to the film, to the author and to the historical and social context in which the work is realised. The director expresses these ideas, especially in *Film Form: Essays in Film Theory and Film Sense* (Eisenstein, 1964). This idea is in line with Vygotsky's ideas that, fully coherent with the Marxist conceptual perspective, placed the entire psychological apparatus of thinking and speech in the vast sea of society and culture dynamics. From a historical perspective, in the post-revolutionary period, there were many Soviet theoreticians who attempted a synthesis of psychology, psychoanalysis, and Marxism. For example, Lev Trotsky in *Literature and Revolution* (1925) wrote:

> The Austrian psycho-analytic school (Freud, Jung, Alfred Adler and others) made an immeasurably greater contribution to the question of the role of sex-element in the forming of individual character and of social consciousness. In fact, there can be no comparison here. Even the most paradoxical exaggerations of Freud are much more significant and fertile than the broad surmises of Rozanov.[1]
>
> *(Trotsky, 1925; Engl. transl., pp. 42, 43)*

In *Problems of Everyday Life* (1923) Trotsky wrote:

> Freud's psychoanalytic approach has a different orientation. It starts with the assumption that the driving force behind the most complex and delicate psychological processes is physiological need. In this general sense he is materialistic, leaving aside the question of whether he does not give undue weight to the sexual factor at the expense of others (this is already a discussion within the confines of materialism). But the psychoanalyst does not face the problems of consciousness in an experimental way, moving from lower to higher phenomena, from simple to complex reflex, but attempts to grasp all these intermediate stages in a single leap, from top to bottom, from religious myth, lyric poem, or dream, directly to the physiological basis of the psyche. Idealists state that the psyche is an independent entity, that the soul is a bottomless pit. Both Pavlov and Freud think that the bottom of the soul is physiology. But Pavlov, like a diver, descends to the bottom and carefully pokes around the well from bottom to top, while Freud stands above the well and with a sharp gaze tries to penetrate its unsettled waters and to catch or glimpse the image of things down below. Pavlov's method is the experiment, Freud's is speculation, sometimes fantastic speculation. The attempt to define psychoanalysis "incompatible" with Marxism and to simply turn one's back to Freudianism is too simple or simplistic. But we are not forced to use Freudianism. It is a work hypothesis that can allow, and certainly allows, deductions and speculations that develop along the line of a materialistic psychology. The experimental procedure will in due course provide verification of these conjectures.
>
> *(Trotsky, 1923; Ital. transl., p. 93)*

In 1910, Trotsky dedicated many pages to Alfred Adler and to his scientific work (Trotsky, 1910). During his stay in Wien, between 1907 and 1914, he personally met the psychoanalyst, Adler, while his wife had become friends with Raissa Adler (see Ellenberger, 1970, p. 585).

This attention of Trotsky's to psychoanalysis placed him in an area regarded with suspicion by regime theorists in the Stalinist period. Aleksandr Etkind dedicated an in-depth study to the relationship between Trotsky and psychoanalysis (see Etkind, 1993, Chapter 7).

Regarding the success of psychoanalysis in the early 1920s, one must remember that a Psychoanalytic Society had been established in Moscow since 1911. It had a short life, but after the war and the revolution, psychoanalysis lived a happy, although brief season in the new Soviet Republic.

In Kazan, where, in 1908, the first Russian Centre of Experimental Psychology was established, a second Psychoanalytic Society was created in 1922 on the initiative of Aleksandr R. Luria, who had studied there. When he moved to Moscow in 1923, after the war and the revolution, Luria made the work of the Muscovite Psychoanalytic Society thrive again.

In Soviet Russia, there had been many attempts, from several perspectives, to create a connection between psychoanalysis and Marxism. The involvement of the Marxist theory was not a due homage or an obligation towards the dominant thought. There was a real interest in psychologists for such a comparison.

In the Soviet science of the time, the distinction between political lines, philosophy, and science was not easy to detect. However, it would be a mistake to interpret the inclusion of Marxism into Soviet psychology of the 1920s because of political pressure. It seems that an opposite spirit animated those who took part in the multiform debate on the future direction of Soviet psychology. There were uncertainties and strong disagreements, but there was also enthusiasm and optimism. In psychology, the initial debate on Marxism, since the 1920s, was characterised by the attempt to merge the two theoretical realities. Scholars explained how their approach to psychology was in tune with Marxist principles. Contact points between Marxism and psychological theory were detected in Kornilov's reactology, Pavlov' and Bekhterev's reflexology, and Luria's psychoanalysis. They all discussed their interdependent nature. Concerning psychoanalysis, among the intellectuals, as Etkin reported "the question of the unconscious 'was for 1920s literature an expression of a general interest in the motive forces of revolution'" (Etkind, 1997, p. 180).

The debate specificity on the relation between psychology and Marxism involved psychologists like Vygotsky and Luria, who had first embraced psychoanalysis and met with the necessity to offer a methodological evaluation, not only of psychoanalytical issues but of psychology in general.

In Moscow, Luria participated in the activity of the Muscovite Psychoanalytic Society; he was the secretary and the founder of a community of psychoanalysts, which was eventually dispersed with the war and the revolution. Vygotsky had actively participated in the meetings and workshops on psychoanalysis. We have records on the activity of both Luria and Vygotsky in the releases sent by Luria to the *Internationale Zeitschrift für Psychanalyse* (Angelini, 1988, p. 114). Luria and Vygotsky participated in the Muscovite Psychoanalytic Society till 1929. The Society was at the heart of Moscow, in the famous "Ryabushinsky House", which also hosted the Psychoanalytic Asylum directed by Vera Schmidt. Among the collaborators there was Sabina Spielrein. At the end of the 1920s, attacks against psychoanalysis heightened and brought to the formal end of society.

In that period, intellectuals involved in artistic production, like Eisenstein, carefully followed the methodological debate, conscious of the fact that their work could gain intellectual consistency, theoretical energy and insights from the ideas raised in that context.

In 1925, the volume *Psychology and Marxism* was published, edited by Konstantin N. Kornilov, and it contained writings by Luria and Vygotsky and other members of the Muscovite Psychoanalytic Society, such as the lawyer M. A. Reisner, the pedagogist P. P. Blonsky, the philosopher B. D. Fridman and the physician A. R. Zalkind. It must be remembered that Blonsky was the promoter of a theoretical idea called "Pedology", which aimed to form and transform human nature in the infantile stage to realise the myth of the Soviet "new man". As stated by Etkind: "Pedology … was founded by people who had gone through relatively serious training in psychoanalysis" (Etkind, 1997, p. 10). The issue of children's and adolescents' education within the domain of a new social project was taken into great account by the Soviet authorities and intellectuals. Tugaybayeva wrote:

> the period was characterized by an upsurge in creativity and relatively free exchange of opinions among the advocates of different theories. Psychoanalysis was being discussed along with reflexology and behavioral research. Advocates of these orientations were forced to readjust to new societal challenges and to the new ideological orientation. Among the questions they had to address concerning their respective approaches were: Does it fall within the spirit of Marxism? Does it permit a materialistic understanding of the world? And, will their orientation help to create the new man conceived of as a builder of communism? Whether or not psychology could even exist within the new ideological context was vigorously debated. Nevertheless, Soviet psychoanalysts energetically started to direct their attention toward research mandated by the new society. One such requirement was the formation of the "new man". From the first days of existence, the Soviet state was concerned with educating children in the spirit of loyalty to the ideas of Bolshevism.
>
> *(Tugaybayeva, 1996, p. 257)*

It is interesting to note that at the end of the 1920s and in the first 1930s, some Soviet psychologists explored the use of cinema as an educational tool. In particular, Gelmont A. Markovich (1895–1963) studied the use of cinema and other media for children's psychological development and school education (see Caroli and Mecacci, 2020, p. 48).

The fields of psychoanalytical interest, investigated by intellectuals involved in this huge scientific and educative enterprise, were extremely wide and theoretically orientated. There were fewer clinical studies, and they were strongly influenced by reflexology, as was the case with the ideas introduced by Zalkind.

Aron Borisovich Zalkind, who was very close to Eisenstein, deserves special attention. He was a crucial figure for a network of psychoanalysts, psychologists, psychiatrists, physicians, and different intellectuals. All these people embraced the ideals of the October Revolution. They considered psychoanalysis a powerful tool to change the world and free men from bourgeois morality. Zalkind faced many difficulties, not only for having embraced psychoanalysis. The main problem he had to tackle was the fact that he was one of the leaders of Soviet pedology, along with the pedagogist Pavel P. Blonsky, also a member of the Muscovite Psychoanalytic Society (Angelini, 1988, pp. 56, 86). Pedology was a psycho-pedagogical movement which spread extensively after the revolution but vanished in the early 1930s, accused of adopting "bourgeoise" ideas and methods. Pedology was banned by a decree of the Central Committee in 1936. After this decree, even the Vygotskyan school was dispersed, as Vygotsky had been one of the leading proponents of pedology and had taught it at the University of Moscow. The very same decree (1946) signed the end of the psychoanalytical movement. In fact, psychoanalysis had been opposed by Stalin's government since 1925. We must wait until 1989 to see Freud's work printed again on Soviet ground.

Zalkind, openly in favour of psychoanalysis, like many other major intellectuals, was the director of the journal *Pedology*, and in 1930, he also became the head of the "Institute of Psychology of Moscow", later renamed "Institute of Psychology, Pedology, and Psychotechnics". Vygotsky and Luria worked in the Institute since 1925.

We have recently learned that Zalkind died in 1936, shortly after the decree. Some people think he had a stroke; others believe he committed suicide (see Mecacci, 2011, p. 102). Eisenstein was introduced to Zalkind in 1923 by Anija Kasatkina, the woman with whom the director had an affair, according to Bulgakova (1998, p. 42). The encounter took place during a representation of his play, *The Wise Man*. After a while, Eisenstein asked Zalkind for a treatment based on psychoanalytical methods. According to Bulgakowa (2001, p. 172), Anya Kasatkina persuaded him to start psychoanalysis to overcome his difficulties with women. Zalkind and the director met several times and did a sort of informal analysis. Zalkind, more Adlerian than Freudian (Mecacci, 2011, p. 102), did not use an orthodox procedure in his treatments. Bulgakova (1998, p. 60) said that it was Zalkind who introduced Eisenstein to Luria and Vygotsky.

Among the main representatives of the pedagogic effort that aimed to give life to "the new man", there was also Pavel P. Blonsky, a member of the Muscovite Psychoanalytic Society and one of the founders of "Pedology". Conceptually, this discipline differed from pedagogy and was at the basis, methodologically, of any pedagogical investigation. The relation between pedology and pedagogy was supposed to be the same as for botanics and gardening. Blonsky, Luria, Vygotsky, Fridman, and many others were researchers at the Moscow State Institute of Experimental Psychology.

This cluster of thinkers mostly addressed controversial and crucial issues of the Marxist theory from a psychoanalytical point of view. They all questioned, from their own perspectives, how the subjective, psychological, individual dimension interacted with the great laws of the social movement described by historical materialism. Eisenstein was concerned with the same issue. In this confrontation, different psychological theories present in Soviet society emerged, such as *Structuralism* with Wundt and Titchener, *Functionalism* with Mead and Thorndike, *Behaviorism* with Wundt, and *Associationism* with Ebbinghaus and Müller. *Associationism* is related to the work of Pavlov and Bekhterev, who took part in the psychological debate from a physiological perspective. Special attention was devoted to *Gestalt*, with Wertheimer, Koffka, Köhler and, later, Lewin. Vygotsky was very interested in the *Gestalt* theory and, with certain critical accents, addressed Lewin's ideas. From April to May 1933, Lewin stayed in Moscow and met Vygotsky; they were friends but also had fruitful intellectual exchanges (see Mecacci, 2017, pp. 130–133).

In post-revolutionary Russia, psychoanalysis successfully spread because it offered useful tools to tackle the relation between the human subject and historical laws. Paradoxically, it was due to this capability and its theoretical connections with Western European Marxist thought – criticised by orthodox Soviets – that psychoanalysis was strongly opposed by theoreticians aligned with official dogmatism.

Vygotsky attracted the attention of Luria and, later, of young Aleksei N. Leontev (1932, 1965, 1977), as he possessed a global conception of the relation between Marxism and psychology. Mecacci wrote:

> According to Vygotsky, in relation to a purely epistemological analysis (the relation theory-methodology, the nature of psychological notions, terminology, etc.) which is valid both for physical and natural sciences, in psychology it is not possible to overlook an examination of the practical applications: from psychopathology and psychotherapy to the extensive range of social sectors which require the use of psychology (from school to work). In this broad vision of psychology, Vygotsky had in mind the perspective chosen by Marx in his critique of political economy. Marx's proposal represented for Vygotsky the most advanced model of psychology investigation, in its complementary dimension, both theoretical and practical. But the reference to Marx was not *directed* to a juxtaposition of psychology and Marxism, mechanically linking ideas of the two instances.
>
> *(Mecacci, 2017, pp. 31, 32)*

This connection will be further investigated, but it is important, at this point, to highlight that, also using the philosophical heritage of Marxism, Vygotsky's approach aimed to point the way to an integral study of the person, both in nature and in society.

In the words of Yaroshevsky,

> Vygotsky belonged to a group of young people (most of them in their twenties and thirties), who surrounded by the total rejection of all existing approaches in the early 1920s, reacted *enthusiastically* to the appeal to recast psychology on the basis of dialectical materialism.
>
> *(Yaroshevsky, 1996, p. 163)*

In fact, at that time, the idea that Marx's and Engels' conceptions could lead to a renovation and to a unique and original perspective within human sciences and art was widely spread among young people. Eisenstein belonged to this group.

As Tugaybayeva recalled, "some investigators engaged in psychoanalytic interpretations of art" (Tugaybayeva, 1996, p. 258) and all, directly or indirectly, dealt with Marxism.

Within this context, Kornilov advanced his notion of "reactology"[2]. The "reaction" was considered the global and articulated set of answers of the organism to the environment.

> The reaction then did not refer to the reflex described by Pavlov or Bekhterev, conceived as an answer to a specific stimulus or to a conditioned or associative well-determined connection. As a global answer of the human organism, the "human reaction" also reflected subjective states and the *inner* motivations determined not only by biological conditions but also by the social and cultural status of the individual.
>
> *(Mecacci, 1976, p. 18)*

However, despite his proposal of an integral psychological approach, within a few years, Kornilov's ideas were strongly criticised. In practice, the experimental aspects of reactology translated into the study of physiological reactions, generally connected to problems of social conditioning, sociocultural context, familiar and school education, work environment, etc. On the other hand, Kornilov used the introspective method – whose scientific value was strongly criticised in those years – to describe the subjective aspects of behavioural reactions. In the wide debate that, since the mid-1920s, intensively questioned the theoretical fundamentals of psychology in the Soviet Union, he faced accusations of dualism and mechanism, which led to the marginalisation of reactological theory although its strong influence on the scientific environment of that period is certain.

The cultural-historical notion developed by Vygotsky in the following years, despite its radical diversity and its critical attitude towards reactology, investigated the same social and historical context to which Kornilov referred. An even stronger influence was found in the research that brought Luria to write *The Nature of Human Conflicts* (1932). With a different theoretical frame, Luria's method of "verbal control of motor behaviour" drew from Kornilov's techniques of motor reaction recording. Eisenstein had the opportunity to witness several experiments that brought Luria to write the volume (see Bulgakova, 1989, p. 84).

With regard to psychoanalytical theories, Kornilov demonstrated, as a matter of fact, an opening towards investigation and confrontation. In the work *Psychology and Marxism,* there were several contributions of exponents of the Russian psychoanalytical movement.

In fact, the Soviet scientific and cultural environment at the beginning of the 1920s was not opposing psychoanalysis. Psychoanalytical thought was, like other ideas, an element which enriched the debate. We can suppose that the novelty of Freudian theories and the light they shed on one of the less studied human characteristics, i.e., sexuality, determined a strong interest in psychoanalysis. One should also consider that several members of the Russian Psychoanalytic Society were sympathisers of Bolshevism or enlisted in the Bolshevik party, such as Aleksandr

Luria, Boris Fridman, Roza Averbuch, Aron Zalkind, and Viktor Kopp. The latter was also sent to Stockholm on diplomatic missions starting in 1929. In the beginning, the comparison between Marxism and psychoanalysis did not see the latter moving from concretely disadvantageous positions.

Moreover, the editions of *Zeitschrift* of that period showed a very lively activity. We could also say that psychoanalysis received a sort of official recognition, within certain limits, with the foundation, in 1922, of the Moscow Psychoanalytic Society by Wulff and Ermakov. Some thinkers believed that Freud's theories could significantly enrich different theoretical fields. Several supporters of psychoanalysis of non-idealist philosophical extraction believed, for instance, that it could provide useful insight into the critique of religious ideology. Such is the case, for example, of Reisner (1924). The critique of religion was the subject of a workshop held by Averbuch, and the issue was further discussed up to 1930 in several meetings of the Psychoanalytic Society. Since 1922, when he was still living in Kazan, Averbuch had shown interest in some possible applications of psychoanalysis in criminal cases and legal proceedings.

Furthermore, Ivan Ermakov and Moshe Wulff belonged to the group of analysts of the Muscovite Psychoanalytic Society. Together with Nikolai Osipov, they translated a great part of Freud's work. Even before the revolution, they had proposed several similarities between art and psychoanalysis. After 1917, they promoted Marxism, even formally, producing several theoretical works and holding public positions in the institutions of the Soviet Republic (see Angelini, 1988, pp. 45, 46). The group was quite large, and the theoretical background extended beyond the context of psychoanalysis to embrace the overall topic of the relation between the human subject and history. In psychology, the interest in Marxism had already been manifested outside Russia for many years. The American psychologist James Mark Baldwin, in *History of Psychology* (1913), stated that under the influence of Marx, the comprehension of the relation between personality – one of the main subjects of psychology – and society had changed.

In Russia, even before the revolution, physiologists like Sechenov, Pavlov, Bekhterev and others had outlined a scientific-natural approach which offered a more acceptable materialistic vision of the subject and its behaviour. This very popular approach was called reflexology. In the Soviet world, it shadowed all the introspective methods used to study personality. Introspective psychology was considered an "ancient fiction" because, from the perspective of reflexologists, it was concerned with a metaphysical entity corresponding to the soul. As Yaroshevsky wrote:

> … in the atmosphere of the early 1920s, characterized by the struggle between reflexology and subjective empirical psychology (and there was no other psychology in Russia at the time), Marxism turned out to be the savior of psychology. Except for its support, psychology would have been swept *away* by the attack of the new credo on what were called ancient fictions.
>
> *(Yaroshevsky, 1996, p. 165)*

Psychoanalysis also played a role in opposing "ancient fiction". As previously mentioned, Averbuch suggested an inquiry into religious ideology, and he analysed some psychoanalytical aspects of a confiscation procedure of church property. The interest of some psychoanalysts regarding legal and criminological issues is not to be underestimated. The years following the revolution had witnessed a rise in criminal actions and juvenile delinquency. Tackling this phenomenon could become a civil commitment, and contributions from psychoanalysis could represent an opportunity for a practical encounter, not only theoretical, between the needs of the new Soviet society and psychoanalytical theory. For example, Reisner, one of the members of the Muscovite Society and with a strong interest in sociological and juridical issues, had presented, in December 1925, a work on "Parasitism and Sexuality" related to prostitution.

In 1926 and 1927, Averbuch and Fridman had become interested in the topic of homosexuality, which had been once again criminalised after the period of relative "sexual liberalisation" described by Reich (1936) after the revolution. Reich himself (1936, p. 171) pointed out that the law did not distinguish among different kinds of homosexuality and highlighted the socially negative aspects of this indiscriminate condemnation.

Vygotsky and Luria met on a regular basis around the mid-1920s with the aim of defining the new Soviet psychology. They were joined shortly after by Leontiev. Cole wrote:

> In the 1920s no Soviet psychologists could ignore Pavlov, though he was by no means accorded for the role of supreme arbiter of Soviet psychology that he would acquire in the 1950s. Rather, the "troika" – as Vygotsky, Luria and Leontiev regarded themselves – accorded Pavlov a restricted role in psychological theory and had the temerity to question the generality of his psychological theory as it applied to integrated behavior. This critical attitude came through clearly in *The Nature of Human Conflicts*, where Aleksandr Romanovich rejected the "telephone switchboard" analogy of the brain, which he identified with Pavlov, opting instead for a "systems' approach" which he identified with Karl Lashley. At the same time, Pavlov's contribution to a physiological theory of the mind was acknowledged, and his experimental studies of conflict and neurosis were important to Aleksandr Romanovich's thinking.
>
> *(Cole, 1979, pp. 205, 206)*

In the beginning, Vygotsky, Luria, and Leontiev continued to work at the Institute of Psychology, directed by Kornilov, speculating on some ideas originating from reactology, also supported by Kornilov. Such a theoretical frame, though, was not satisfying for them. When their own thoughts began to emerge, they, too, left the Institute. In 1927–1928, even though they still were associated with Kornilov's institute, Vygotsky, Luria, and Leontiev joined the *Psychological Laboratory* of the Academy of *Communist Education*. Vygotsky became also involved in the organisation of the Institute of Defectology, which had at its core the research on the development of mentally disabled children. Besides a formulation and review of the contemporary school of psychology critical thinking, the *troika* began to train students according to their own thoughts and research lines. While they reached the conclusion that their new theory required new methods, they gathered around them a small but enthusiastic group of students with the aim of starting new experimentations. That is how the *pyatorka* (or group of five students) was formed, a cluster which included Lidiya I. Bozhovich, In Roza E. Levina, Natalya G. Morozova, Liya S. Slavina, and Aleksandr Zaporozhets. Some of these scholars, who were tutored by Luria, became prominent figures of Soviet psychology after the Second World War.

It is important to mention the name of Zaporozhets (1905–1981), an exceptional figure who was both Sergei Eisenstein's student and friend. In the words of Cole:

> [Luria] and Vygotsky, for example, met regularly with Sergei Eisenstein to discuss the ways in which the abstract ideas that formed the core of historical materialism could be embodied in visual images projected upon the movie screen. By happenstance Zaporozhets, who had been an actor in the Ukraine before going to Moscow and had been recommended to Sergei Eisenstein, eventually ended up a psychologist. At the end of the 1920s he played the role of psychology's 'ear' in the world of the film, attending Eisenstein's discussion, which he reported to Vygotsky and Luria. Eisenstein enlisted his psychologist friends' help in solving not only the difficult problem of translation between verbal and visual concepts but also the empirical problem of assessing success. With their aid he constructed *questionnaires* for audiences composed variously of students, workers, and peasants, to determine if they had understood his images as he intended.
>
> *(Cole, 1979, p. 207)*

For Vygotsky and Luria, there was a significant connection between the child's cognitive development, which they defined as the cultural development of the child and the evolution of human culture. The same issue is outlined in *Human Conflicts* (Luria, 1932).

In fact, the analogy between cultural evolution and individual development belonged, in an intrinsic way, to the evolutive psychology of the first years of the twentieth century. The analogy is clearly outlined in the works by Lucien Lévy Bruhl, which attracted Eisenstein's interest and significantly influenced Piaget and the German evolutive psychologist Heinz Werner. Vygotsky and Luria had known them since the 1920s. This approach was in line with the general idea supported by the *troika*, i.e., development is characterised by the evolution of more and more complex forms of mediated behaviour. Vygotsky and Luria published further observations on the evolutive analogy in *Studies on the History of Behavior: Ape, Primitive, and Child* (1930).

From a wider perspective, within Marxist thought, a special sensibility towards the problem of the relation between the "subjective human factor" and social context had developed, especially in the German and Austrian cultural left wing since the beginning of the century. This particular interest continued to be nourished in different forms till the rise of Nazism.

After the October Revolution, this topic also drew the attention of the less dogmatic theoretical milieus of Soviet society and, historically, conditioned the position of psychoanalysis in the general debate. In the beginning, these ideas emerged, in the years before the First World War, in the movement known as Austro-Marxism, a stream of thought born in Austria, aimed to review some Marxist ideas.

It was difficult to understand wide and complex events such as the war, the October Revolution, nationalist sentiments, the failed Western revolutions, and Nazism itself. In such manifestations, the "subjective human factor" was dominant. The irrational features of these events were not to be explained only by using classical categories of "scientific Marxism", devoid of sufficient insights into the subject's psychological reality. In those years, among different Marxist intellectuals, including Soviet ones, emerged the revaluation of human activity in its various aspects, including the subjective, or rather, the psychological.

I limit myself, in this context, to some explicative indications to better understand how the debate on the "subjective factor" and its relationship with psychoanalysis could have influenced and generated conflicts in the cultural context in which the interest of Eisenstein towards psychoanalysis emerged.

In the first years of the century, the Austrian socialist Max Adler had offered an interesting insight on the topic of "subjective factor" in the work *Causality and Teleology in the Fight for Science* (1904). He aimed, in the perspective of a non-gross Marxism, to the foundation of a "Marxist psychology", which was the same objective eventually pursued by many Soviet psychologists. His ideas connected any social phenomenon to human action. Within this perspective, he addressed the issue of "unconscious motivation". Max Adler was, presumably, influenced by the psychoanalyst Alfred Adler, who, in 1909, had introduced the issue of the relation between Marx and Freud during meetings of the Wien Psychoanalytic Society.

On a philosophical level, the ideas of Adler kept a polemical autonomy with respect to Freudian doctrine. He claimed that the Freudian doctrine made the mistake of having given instincts too wide a role with concern to phenomena of psychological and social life, which were characterised, in his opinion, by a prevalence of sociological contents. Later, in the work *Grundlegung der materialistischen Geschichtsauffassung = Lehrbuch Der materialistischen Geschichtsauffassung* (1930), he shared with other thinkers of his time, for example, Wilhelm Reich (1933a, 1933b), the idea that Communism and primitive matriarchy were replaced by social class division, due to the irruption of patriarchal society. Among the vivid ideas that spread after the October Revolution, many intellectuals and psychologists believed that psychoanalysis could offer the basis for developing Marxist psychological thought.

Psychoanalysis represented the missing element between structure and superstructure, dominated by the human psyche, against any automatic reading of historical events, as suggested by "mechanistic Marxism". To have a scientific validation, psychoanalysis needed to be rooted in a materialistic epistemology.

Luria's works *Psychoanalysis in Light of the Principal Tendencies in Contemporary Psychology* (1923) and *Psychoanalysis as a System of Monistic Psychology* (1925) move towards this direction, giving a crucial role, in a Marxist sense, to psychoanalytical ideas. It was Miller who highlighted the epistemological features in this last work by Luria. According to this perspective, Marxism

> assumed the world to be 'a single system of material processes,' devoid of dualism and of nonmaterialist and static phenomena. In terms of psychology, this translated into the postulate that 'the human mind is a product of the brain and in the final analysis, of the effects of the social *environment* and the class relations and conditions production underlying it on the brain and on each individual human being'.
>
> *(Miller, 1998, p. 80)*

The very aim was to put an end to the mind-body dualism. Later, in Western Europe, the subject was discussed by some psychanalysts with a Marxist orientation, sensitive to the Soviet cultural and scientific debate.

Wilhelm Reich wrote *Dialectical Materialism and Psychoanalysis* (1929), while Otto Fenichel published *Psychoanalysis as the Nucleus of a Future Dialectical* (1934), and both had been influenced by Luria's ideas, even if they elaborated them in different ways (see Angelini, 1996, 2008).

On a strictly philosophical level and in the same years, Gyorgy Lukacs – within a theoretical matrix of Hegelian derivation, which was very different from the Kantian conceptual background of Max Adler – aimed to re-evaluate the ethical dimension suggested in *History and Class Conscience* (1923), precisely to bring historical events back to human actions. It is important to note that the individual psychological issue was always detached from the theoretical domain of Lukacs, who was against any possible integration of Marxism with psychology and psychoanalysis. The subject analysed by Lukacs is always a social and historical subject.

In the same period, Karl Korsch introduced his theories, and in *Marxism and Philosophy* (1923), he developed ideas on the relation between practice and consciousness, criticising Marxist ideas which, according to him, reduced historical materialism to a merely economic notion. On a philosophical level, Korsch highlighted that the "reversal" of the Hegelian dialectic made by Marxism could not simply translate into replacing ideas with the matter. In this, he opposed the mechanistic objectivism promoted by different theoreticians of the Second International, such as Karl Kautsky, who suggested a deterministic notion of history, underestimating subjective elements. In general, the issue of a revaluation of human practice and consciousness in those years spread among the left wing of the Austrian and German communists.

Among these communist thinkers, belonging or about to belong to the so-called Austro-Marxist area echoed theoretical issues which were also alive in the Soviet world.

In the Soviet context, people of culture and researchers belonging to different fields, like Eisenstein, Vygotsky and Luria, believed that psychology and psychoanalysis could offer significant answers on where to position "subjective factor" within the conceptual frame of Marxism.

In this situation, in the Muscovite intellectual domain, there were two factions, openly in favour of or opposed to the hypothesis of a connection between Marxism and psychoanalysis. Unfortunately, the supporters of psychoanalysis were significantly disadvantaged by the fact that the dogmatic Soviet theoreticians located psychoanalysis between the conceptual area of Austro-Marxism and Trotsky's ideas. It was a cluster of ideas heavily criticised by those who, right or wrong, wanted to defend the purity of dialectical materialism. Thus, every thought on psychoanalysis and in general on the "subjective factor" and the psychological dimension in general was historically harshly criticised by the supporters of the official doctrinal Marxist system.

In fact, the attack on psychoanalysis was led by two Soviet theoreticians, Vladimir Iurinets in *Psychoanalyse und Marxismus* (1925) and Deborin in *G. Lukacs and his Criticism of Marxism* (1924). The attack was carried out by the German August Thalheimer who, in *Die Auflösung des Austromarxismus* (1926), was harshly critical towards Max Adler.

Montani observed that Eisenstein "anticipates ideas that the Marxist considerations on art and aesthetics achieved only many years later, for example, in the last works of Lukacs" (1981, p. XIV).

As a matter of fact, observant intellectuals did not consider psychoanalysis as the main enemy of the regime; their aim was to defend the materialist dialectics against mechanistic Marxism;

> For their part, Marxist Soviet theoreticians like Iurinets and Deborin - committed to defend dialectics from the attacks of the mechanist - reacted to the re-evaluation of the subjective factor as a further attack to the dialectic from a different angle. In this vivid controversy, psychoanalysis was also involved, as an overt expression of an interest towards individual subjectivity.
>
> *(Angelini, 1988, p. 190)*

To paraphrase, "the baby was thrown out with the bathwater". Russian psychoanalysts had tried to face the criticism, also on a philosophical level, through several works. Fridman, in January 1924, with a presentation titled "Contribution to the Psychology of Idealism" (see Marti, 1976; Ital. transl., 1978, p. 138) had even tried to give a psychoanalytical interpretation of the idealist theoretical perspective. But it is on the ground of a confrontation between Marxism and psychoanalysis that the most interesting contributions were written and which stimulated debate.

In the Spring of 1925, a public debate on the topic of "Psychoanalysis and Marxism" was held at the "Press Centre" in Moscow. The debate went on for two evenings, gathering a large audience. In the same year, Iurinets published an article criticising psychoanalytical ideas in the magazine *Unter dem Banner des Marxismus* (1925) and expressed several ideas against the possibility of a connection between psychoanalysis and Marxism. Many replied against this position: Wulff, Reisner, Charasov, W. Rohr, Luria, Schaffiz, Fridman, Vhukov, and Zalkind. As Marti stated, they counterattacked Iurinets by saying that they were the ideas of "all of them" (Marti, 1976, p. 140).

In the following years, rejection towards psychoanalysis became official. In the words of Tugaybayeva:

> In 1931, Stalin published his letter titled 'Notes on the History of Bolshevism' in the journal *Proletarskaia Revolyutsia*. He referred to Trotskyism as 'a vanguard of the counterrevolutionary bourgeoisie' and called for a bitter struggle against 'rotten liberalism' and 'Trotskyite contraband' … After that, the movement against psychoanalysis turned into a persecution of 'class enemies in science'. A search for enemies who brought the Trotskyite contraband into the Soviet Union was initiated. The first issue of *Psichologia*, published in 1932, carried articles of Talankin, Shemiakin and Gershonovich, who said that they had identified a direct link between psychoanalysis and Trotskyism … Trotsky was portrayed as the ideological advocate for psychoanalysis and an opponent of materialism and Marxism. Those who accepted Freud and found in psychoanalysis ideas compatible with the Marxist view of psychology were automatically included in the category of Trotskyite contraband… Early in 1931, a series of meetings was held in the Academy of Communist Education wherein the 'the ideological mistake' of Luria, Vygotsky, Zalkind, and others were pointed out. They were said to have exhibited 'a casual attitude' toward psychoanalysis and Freudianism … In the press and academic circles, public retractions of "ideologically incorrect visions" were demanded. Those who had been associated with psychoanalysis had to confess their past mistakes and sins, then acknowledge that the orientation was 'a biological, anti-Marxist and reactionary' theory.
>
> *(Tugaybayeva, 1996, p. 263)*

This schematically sketched scenario helps to understand the theoretical reasons that swiped psychoanalysis away from the Soviet cultural world, forcing personalities such as Vygotsky and Luria to abandon the psychoanalytical point of view on a theoretical level. In 1940, Luria wrote the entry "Psychoanalysis" for the *Soviet Encyclopaedia*. As Miller recalls, Luria wrote:

> Freud had then moved from his early clinically based explorations into the theoretical speculations of "metapsychology", in which he sought to explain large-scale phenomena such as religion, war, and the organization of society in

> terms of universal patterns of aggression, hostility and repression … some of his objections to Freud's ideas would appear decades later in Western critiques of psychoanalysis, stripped of the ideological framework which Luria was obliged to heed.
>
> *(Miller, 1998, p. 108)*

It would be worth mentioning sociological considerations, but they are beyond the scope of the present work and concern the historical meaning of the political storm that, with Stalin, impacted the Soviet Union. It was in this situation, conflictual and problematic, that Eisenstein approached psychoanalytical notions and wanted, somehow, to use them to elaborate his idea of the arts.

Notes

1 Vasilij V. Rozanov (1856–1919) was a proponent of a sort of naturalistic religion of sex and procreation.

2 See K. N. Kornilov (1930), "Psychology in the Light of Dialectic Materialism", in C. Murchison (ed.), *Psychologies of 1930*, Worcester, MA: Clark University Press, pp. 243–278, 1930; K. N. Kornilov (1922), *Uchenie o reaktsiyach cheloveka (Reaktologiya)* [Theory of Human Reactions (Reactology)], Moscow: Gosizdat, Moscow; K. N. Kornilov (ed.) (1925), *Psychologiya i marksizm* (Psychology and Marxism), Moscow: Gosizdat.

3

MARXISM AND PSYCHE

The main contribution of Marx to psychology is related to his idea that the psyche is subordinated to actual life. In the notion of psyche, we must include all the higher psychological functions and – firstly – the process of knowledge. Alexei Leontiev, a psychologist who began his activity collaborating with Vygotsky, wrote: "Cognition does not exist outside the life process that in its very nature is a material, practical process" (Leontiev, 1977; Engl. transl., p. 45). This idea should not be considered obvious because – historically – it was often missing in the field of psychology on an epistemological level.

Nevertheless, independently from Marxism, this perspective – which has independent philosophical foundations – appeared in a psychological and neurological domain – in twentieth-century Positivism. This viewpoint is also implicit in the way Freud looked at cerebral and psychological organisation, as he stated:

> In the first place, our organization – that is, our mental apparatus – has been developed precisely in the attempt to explore the external world, and it must therefore have realized in its structure some degree of expediency; in the second place, it is itself a constituent part of the world which we set out to investigate, and it readily admits of such an investigation; thirdly, the task of science is fully covered if we limit it to showing how the world must appear to us in consequence of the particular character of our investigation; fourthly, the ultimate findings of science, precisely because of the way in which they are acquired, are determined not only by our organization but by the things *which* have affected that organization; finally, the problem of the nature of the world without regard to our percipient mental apparatus is an empty abstraction, devoid of practical interest.
>
> *(Freud, 1927; Engl. transl., pp. 55, 56)*

DOI: 10.4324/9781003398554-4

Of course, one should not confuse these Freudian insights, influenced by nineteenth-century positivist materialism, with the ideas fostered by people like Leontiev, who developed their own general "Theory of Activity" in line with Marxism thought.

Historically, one could stereotypically think that the interest in Marxism of Soviet scientists – psychoanalysts included –was a due passage. According to this opinion, in advancing any proposal, intellectuals and scientists first had to pay tribute to the "founding fathers" of the revolution and then express their ideas. Paradoxically, this could create the opposite effect and suggest that the Marxist philosophical framework was irrelevant compared to the actual work of intellectuals and scientists, psychologists, and psychoanalysts.

Certainly, there were situations in the history of the Soviet Union in which this was true, but it is wrong to generalise. One should not underestimate the genuine commitment of that generation of intellectuals and scholars who searched, within the Marxist dialectical philosophy, epistemological assurances in support of their own scientific work. In those years, before any other period, the complexity of the relation among psychology, psychoanalysis, and philosophical innovations was deeply investigated.

Even intellectuals like Vygotsky and Luria, regardless of pressure, wanted to develop their ideas in harmony with the political and philosophical trends of that period. As happened with Eisenstein, they acknowledged dialectical philosophy as a guarantee of validity for their ideas. Philosophy, science and politics clearly appeared to be connected. Deploying dialectical materialism to address their intellectual enterprises was, for the October Revolution generation, a most needed and inevitable choice.

Marxism was interpreted as the theory capable of offering the highest guarantees of method to face the wide repertoire of human science and politics thanks to both Lenin's methodological and philosophical work, *Materialism and Empirio-Criticism* (1909) and the publication of Engels' *Dialectics of Nature* (1925).

These realities wanted to be transferred from the world of ideal aspirations of the Romantic Age to the twentieth-century scientific dimension, and Marxism seemed to be able to make this passage possible. In those years, intellectuals wondered whether the encounter between psychological theory and psychoanalysis with Marxism would be able to generate a new kind of research and create the foundations of a completely new approach to psychology. Within this context, Vygotsky's ideas emerged and assumed great relevance.

Vygotsky claimed that, using Marxist principles, a new kind of psychology was possible. The debate first involved Marxist psychologists that were confronted with the necessity to offer an evaluation not only of the notion of conscious and psychoanalytical issues but of psychology itself. In this perspective, we should look at the volume *Psychology and Marxism*, edited by Kornilov in 1925. The volume, as Kornilov stated in the premise, was the "result of a collective work of the collaborators of the Muscovite Centre of Experimental Psychology" (Kornilov, 1925), and it tackled general issues connected to the relation between Marxism and psychology. This direction was already clearly reflected in the titles of some articles, for example, the ones by Luria and Fridman. Luria proposed *Psychoanalysis as a System of Monist Psychology* (1925), and Fridman *The Main Psychological Notions of Freud and the Theory of Historical Materialism* (1925). Vygotsky presented *Consciousness as a Problem in the Psychology of Behaviour* (1925a), wherein he quotes Freud's *The Ego and the Id* (1922). Reisner contributed to the general debate with *Social Psychology and Marxism* (1925a) and Blonsky with *Psychology as a Science of Behaviour Science* (1925). In the same year, Reisner also published *Social Psychology and Freud's Doctrine* (1925b), a work that, through psychoanalysis, presented several sociological and political considerations. Kornilov, who had become director of the Institute of Experimental Psychology of Moscow in 1923, titled the volume with his opening essay, getting to the core of the problem. He had already expressed the need for an anti-spiritualist, Marxist, and concrete psychology during the first pan-Russian Conference on Psychoneurology in January 1924. In his speech, he shed light on materialism in psychology, claiming the non-substantial distinctiveness between psyche and matter. Compared to the classical solutions that suggested either psychophysics parallelism or the interaction between the two elements, Kornilov introduced the notions of function and functional localisation. He criticised the empirical psychology of nineteenth-century tradition, defining it with a term also used by Luria, "mosaic psychology". He also criticised some theories by Pavlov and Bekhterev, which, according to him, were unable to grasp the historical, social, and cultural conditions – which determine higher psychological processes – in physiological terms. He thus suggested an "integral approach" (Kornilov, 1925) to human behaviour.

Cole wrote:

> The volume *Psychology and Marxism*, edited by Kornilov in 1925, reveals the difference between Aleksandr Romanovich's and Vygotsky's approaches at the time. Luria's Marxism was based on the peripheral Marxist writings with obvious psychological implications, such as Marx's *Theses on Feuerbach* or *Engels' Anti-Dühring*. Vygotsky began with *Das Capital*. When Engel's *Dialectics of Nature* appeared in 1925, Vygotsky immediately incorporated it into his thinking. Whatever other shortcomings Vygotsky's thinking may have had, opportunistic parroting of Marxism was not one of them.
>
> *(Cole, 1979, p. 204)*

Soviet intellectuals engaged in human sciences looked at the ideas of Marx and Lenin as a methodological instrument which would prevent them from falling into pure ideology. The term ideology referred to notions that, according to Marxists, were, in the last analysis, *opinions*, sometimes even culturally relevant, but without actual foundations and thus considered subjective and controversial. It was Boris Fridman who tackled a classical question related to the debate on Marxism, psychoanalysis, and psychology: "what are the mechanisms of the formation of an ideology?" Or, more specifically, what is the 'connecting link' between economic-social reality and the ideologies in the psyche? Differently from Reich, who – with in the 1930s – connected family (a precise sociological entity) to the mechanism of reproduction of the dominant ideology, Fridman addressed the problem through more speculative notions. In his work *The Main Psychological Notions of Freud and the Theory of Historical Materialism* (1925), he introduced the notion of rationalisation to explain the ways ideologies were formed. One only needs to remember that psychoanalysis, with the term rationalisation, refers to the process through which the individual tends to explain in a logically coherent and morally acceptable way a behaviour, an action, an idea, a feeling or other, without perceiving the actual reasons. More specifically, it refers to the rationalisation of a symptom, of a defensive coaction or a reactive formation. Despite its apparent defensive function, rationalisation is not generally classified as a defensive mechanism. In fact, it is not directly oriented against the fulfilment of drives, but it is deployed to disguise – secondarily – the actual aspect of the defensive conflict. Freud associated it with the mechanism of secondary elaboration, i.e., the procedure which places dream images in a coherent scenario. Not only political theories and cultural conventions were considered ideologies, but also different religions. The premise of these assumptions was the idea that, in the Marxist method, a "scientific" perspective existed also in social and cultural domains. In the name of this scientific aspiration – or at least of epistemological correctness – the ideology, in all its diverse expressions, had to be subjected to a theoretical and methodological analysis.

In the context of human sciences, the so-called "science of the soul" of nineteenth-century derivation, the risk of falling into the opinability was, and still is the main threat. Young people who had actively participated in the October Revolution had rejected past ideologies and opinions. Marxism represented a method capable of attaching hopefully scientific validity to psychological and sociological notions, which also belonged to domains not close to exact sciences. Following this direction in the field of art, Eisenstein believed that methodological criteria deriving from Marxism could provide a theoretical framework which invested his own conceptual proposals with validity beyond ideologies and opinions.

Vygotsky, who was a friend of Eisenstein and a reference point for psychology, had introduced new ideas which aimed to be organised according to the criteria of scientific realism. For Eisenstein, these theoretical criteria, which derived from the Marxist theoretical background, could provide veridical contributions also to speculations around art and cinema. In some circumstances, the director referred to the words of Lenin and Engels as existential references (see page 78 of this volume). To evaluate the methodological meaning that the ideas of Marx and Lenin historically assumed, we should consider not only the theoretical framework but also the emotional involvement of the young Soviet intellectuals.

Starting from Marx, it is possible to outline, a stream of thought related to individual psychological problems. Marx, as it is known, believed that dominant relations of production and the subsequent social relations within which human existence unfolds were prior to the formation of the individual psyche; he thus stated that there was a primacy of social dynamics over the psyche. This idea is expressed in several works by Marx in a systematic way. In *The Economic and Philosophic Manuscripts of 1844*, Marx states:

> We see how the history of *industry* and the established *objective* existence of industry are the *open* book of *man's essential powers*, the exposure to the senses of human *psychology*. Hitherto this was not conceived in its inseparable connection with man's *essential being*, but only in an external relation of utility, because, moving in the realm of estrangement, people could only think of a man's general mode of being – religion or history in its abstract-general character as politics, art, literature, etc. – as the reality of man's essential powers and *man's species activity*. We have before us the *objectified essential powers* of man in the form of *sensuous, alien, useful objects*, in the form of estrangement, displayed in *ordinary material industry* (which can be conceived as well as a part of that general movement, just that movement can be conceived as a *particular* part of industry, since all human activity hitherto has been labor – that is, industry – activity estranged from itself). A *psychology* for which this, the part of history most contemporary and accessible to sense, remains a closed book, cannot become a genuine, comprehensive and *real* science. What indeed are we to think of a science which *airily* abstracts from this large part of human labor, and which fails to feel its own incompleteness, while such a wealth of human endeavor, unfolded before it, means nothing more to it than, perhaps, what can be expressed in one word, "need", "*vulgar need*"? […] *Industry* is the *actual*, historical relationship of nature, and therefore of natural *science*, to man. If, therefore, industry is conceived as the *exoteric* revelation of man's *essential powers*, we also gain an understanding of the *human* essence of nature or the *natural* essence of man.
>
> *(Marx, 1844; Engl. transl., pp. 142, 143)*

Even better known are some passages in the *German Ideology*:

> … we do not set out from what men say, imagine, conceive, nor from men as narrated, thought of, imagined, conceived, in order to arrive at men in the flesh. We set out from real, active men, and on the basis of their real life-process we demonstrate the development of the ideological reflexes and echoes of this life-process. The phantoms formed in the human brain are also, necessarily, sublimates of their material life-process, which is empirically verifiable and bound to material premises. Morality, religion, metaphysics, all the rest of *ideology* and their corresponding forms of consciousness, thus no longer retain the semblance of independence. […] Life is not determined by consciousness, but consciousness by life.
>
> *(Marx and Engels, 1846, first published in full in 1932; Engl. transl., pp. 14, 15)*

The list of topics related to psychology and discussed by Marx and Engels is definitively rich, but it suffices for the scope of the present work to underline the historical value of their speculations in comparison to the subsequent development of Lenin's ideas, which represented a reference for young intellectuals, Eisenstein included.

Although he never directly discussed the context of psychological issues, Lenin dedicated a significant part of his intellectual work to the analysis of problems connected to the development of science in his time. Within this context and within even wider theoretical levels, Lenin addressed the analysis of philosophical issues related to the theme of knowledge and to the relation between individual and the world, expressing several relevant ideas for the notion of the psyche and Soviet psychology.

The main work in which such topics are examined is *Materialism and Empirio-Criticism* (1909). Similar topics are tackled in other works, particularly *Philosophical Books*, published in 1929–1930, after his death.

To understand the importance of the psychological ideas expressed by Lenin in *Materialism and Empirio-Criticism*, it is necessary to contextualise the reasons why the work was written. Since the beginning of the century, Empirio-Criticism had entered Russian philosophy and science and was considered the ultimate intellectual trend in European culture. This philosophy was connected to Mach, Avenarius, Poincaré, Duhem, and Ostwald, the promoters of Energeticism. Empirio-criticism thinkers were commonly referred to as "machists".

In 1905, in Russia, there was a revolutionary outburst, which was settled within a few months. Lenin had secretly reached Peterburg in October 1905, but at the end of December, he was forced to leave the country. In the period following this failed revolution, the empirio-criticist approach had widely spread within the Russian social democracy. In the general upheaval of political movements after 1905, Empirio-Criticism gathered much interest because it addressed problems not directly connected to action and because the critical drive it displayed seemed very useful for a philosophical rethinking.

In the arts, a relevant figure of this philosophy was Aleksandr A. Bogdanov, founder of the Proletkult, where Eisenstein worked (in the drama division) at the time of *Montage of Attractions*. Bogdanov significantly influenced the Soviet artistic avant-garde and the film industry (see Montani, 1975).

Lenin considered the presence of Empirio-Criticism like an ideological drift in socialism and manifested a political and theoretical concern because many "machists" sought a synthesis between this philosophy and Marxism, believing this would "modernise" Marxist concepts.

Moreover, on a political level, Lenin had strong disagreements with the "machists" on how to judge the consequences of the failed democratic revolution of 1905. The machists, among other things, in contrast to Lenin and following the dissolution of the achievements of that revolution, demanded the immediate withdrawal of the Social Democratic deputies from the State Duma.

To understand the reasons that led Lenin to oppose machists' ideas, it is necessary to introduce, synthetically, the two different notions of materialism and Empirio-criticism.

From a philosophical point of view, we can define materialist as any philosophy that indisputably accepts the existence of the world independently from its interactions with mankind. In this perspective, the ideal totality of natural facts is considered like the set of elements of a primitive matter conceived both in a static sense and in motion, consequently subject to changes in form. The origin of man is thus connected to matter in motion, in its highest form of organisation.

Nevertheless, human feelings do not represent an indissoluble ensemble with the other parts of matter. In fact, these feelings are triggered by the encounter of the physiological structure of the individual with pre-existing and external objects.

The consequence is that, clearly, these objects can exist independently from the existence of a human being who comes to know them. Epicureus is the philosopher who most mirrors materialism. According to him, human life is the result of atomic aggregates in motion, and feelings are mechanical relations among different so-called atoms of the soul and objects. Epicurean ideas played an important role in Marx's education.

Very different from materialism is the sensist perspective, connected to Empirio-Criticism. We can synthetically say that according to the sensist perspective, human knowledge develops from sensations. From a certain point of view, it seems that sensism can be associated with materialism. It shares with it the critique towards preliminary and innate notions which regulate human cognitive processes. As it considers sensations a "primum", sensism can turn into agnosticism, a perspective which was strongly opposed by Lenin.

Empirio-criticism can be included in sensism, even though this identification requires some clarifications. Regardless of the nuances of the different representatives, it is understood that Empirio-criticism is a philosophy which supports the unity of experience, deleting any metaphysical dichotomy between subject and object. There is no fundamental difference between psychological and physical knowledge and matter. Nevertheless, because sensations were not considered observations of what is external to the subject but like inseparable elements from what provoked them, it is not possible, according to Lenin, to attribute to Empirio-Criticism the notion of a matter prior to the human subject. Of course, both Mach and Avenarius admitted the existence of biological organisms in geological periods prior to the present age, with cognitive mechanisms different from our own. But, as they did not consider the world as an external entity compared to the sentient subject, it was possible to detect the possibility, polemically and ironically underlined by Lenin (1909, Chapters 1 and 5), that before the appearance of the human species on earth, the image of the planet and the planet itself were radically different, coherent with the sensations perceived by prehuman organisms.

Leaving aside an evaluation of this conclusion, we must admit that the empirio-criticist position originated from the wish to reconcile the value of Kantian thought with the philosophical importance of sciences. In fact, to a first materialistically oriented interpretation, Kant's thought would seem incompatible with a scientific vision of the world. According to Kant, knowledge is limited to the realm of experience. Moreover, in this realm, we cannot know the "thing in itself", the so-called *noumena*, but only the way things present themselves as *a priori* forms of reason. In other words, we know things as *phenomena*.

On the contrary, according to scientific materialist thought, any science which cannot assert an effective coincidence between facts and images is devoid of meaning. It is worth underlining that even those who, since the last century, authoritatively supported Leninist ideas were not particularly worried to emphasise Lenin's philosophical rigour (see Geymonat, 1972, pp. 105, 106). Rather, they were more concerned about clarifying the concrete importance of reasons that made him reject machists' ideas.

Lenin was afraid that the philosophical weight of the cognitive value of sciences was directly and seriously threatened by the empirio-criticist theses. Empirio-Criticism, in the effort to reconcile Kantianism and Materialism, ultimately reduced sensations and the causes of sensations into a single unity. One should also consider that the historical period was characterised by a significant crisis of the sciences. The nineteenth-century scientific discoveries, like thermodynamic and electromagnetism theory, had undermined the mechanist's asset of science, which underwent violent shocks with the scientific progress of the first twentieth century. It is obvious that, for methodological reasons, the problem of the relationship between the external world and the psyche was very much present in Soviet psychology and psychoanalysis.

In the analysis of the conceptual contents of that period, the ideas of Engels and Lenin surface in many contexts. With concern to psychology, Lenin found good feedback to his ideas in the reflexological work of Ivan Pavlov, although Pavlov's methodologies were different from Lenin's. In fact, Lenin's ideas significantly impacted, theoretically, Soviet psychology as they tackled, directly aspects related to *perception* and *cognition*. It is thus useful to carry a brief review of Lenin's ideas, summing them up in the following points:

I *Reflection theory*. Having assumed the objectivity of the external world, the reflection takes place, initially, in relation to sensorial knowledge and then extends to all kinds of knowledge. In the words of Lenin, reflection is "the recognition of real objects outside us, to which our conceptions 'correspond'" (Lenin, 1909; Engl. transl., p. 80); and furthermore: "[For materialism] the fundamental belief is that outside of us and independently of us, there exist objects, things, and bodies; that our perception is images of the outer world" (Lenin, 1909; Engl. transl., p. 78). Lenin also stated that: "Matter is a philosophic category that refers to the objective reality given to man in his sensations – a reality which is copied, photographed, and reflected by our sensations, but which exists independently of them" (Lenin, 1909; Engl. transl., pp. 101, 102). In a way, these Leninist ideas represent hypotheses with a physiological background concerning the functioning of perceptive psychological functioning. From a wider perspective, they clearly express the generality of a philosophical attitude. The notion of reflex strongly influenced Soviet psychology, playing the role of an epistemological discriminant.

II *Relativity of Knowledge*. According to it, scientific knowledge, while approximating reality, can never offer a complete depiction of it. As Lenin avers:

> From the standpoint of modern materialism, or Marxism, the relative limits of our approximation to the cognition of the objective, *absolute* truth are historically conditioned, but the existence of this truth is unconditioned, as well as the fact contestable that we are continually approaching it ... The materialistic dialectic of Marx and Engels certainly does contain relativism, but it is not reduced to it, that is, it recognises the relativity of all our knowledge, not in the sense of the denial of objective truth, but in the sense of the historical conditions which determine the degrees of our knowledge as it approaches this truth.
>
> *(Lenin, 1909; Engl. transl., p. 136)*

III *Thesis of deepening (of knowledge)*, i.e., the idea that the succession of one scientific theory to another (e.g., from twentieth-century physics to nineteenth-century mechanism) does not depend on their conventionality, but rather on the deepening of knowledge achieved by the new theories, compared to the previous ones.

IV *The criterion of practice*, i.e., the necessity to keep together theory and practice, as the practice allows the assessment of theoretical results: "Things exist outside of us. Our perceptions and representations are their images. The verification over these images, the distinction of true and false images is given by practice" (Lenin, 1909; Engl. transl., p. 83).

V *Non-definitive proof*. According to this idea, our knowledge is always open to new investigations. In the words of Lenin:

> Of course, we must not forget that the criterion of practice, in the nature of things, neither confirms nor refutes completely any human presentation. This criterion is sufficiently indefinite not to allow human knowledge to become "absolute", and at the same time sufficiently definite to wage a bitter struggle with all varieties of idealism and agnosticism.
>
> *(Lenin, 1909; Engl. transl., p. 114).*

From what has been briefly outlined above, a conception of consciousness emerges that transcends the limits of the philosophical programme and possesses strong psychological values. This perspective is suitable for the use of psychology within the scientific and social debate.

The problem Lenin addressed in *Materialism and Empirio-Criticism*, in philosophical terms, implied essential political issues. Empirio-Criticism was a philosophy tuned with nineteenth-century Positivism. Lenin's work aimed to provide a dialectical answer to the mechanistic and reductionist statements of the nineteenth century. As a matter of fact, Lenin supported Pavlov and his work. Without denying the great scientific value of Pavlov's theories, it would be a paradox to imagine Pavlov's theory as a contribution to a dialectical philosophical perspective. Pavlov's work represented the most significant attempt, in the first half of the twentieth century, to elaborate a theory of behaviour on physiological foundations. It is a classic example of physiological reductionism, inherited by nineteenth-century Positivism. Reductionism is a scientific methodology according to which the phenomena of different "sectors" of reality are connected by a certain order, almost layered. Therefore, facts of a given sector can be "reduced" and explained according to the laws of science investigating the underlying sector. At the basis of this idea, there is physics, most specifically mechanics. In this perspective, sociological phenomena must be interpreted in psychological terms, psychological phenomena in biological terms, biological phenomena in chemical terms, chemical phenomena in physical terms and the latter in mechanic terms. Such apparent guarantees of "scientificity", mechanistically based, are very distant from the dialectical philosophical perspective, which describes, philosophically, the reciprocal action of one or more forces within a system. From a Marxist perspective, such forces can be natural or social. They can also be concepts or ideas. These forces meet and interconnect and eventually get transformed, even clashing and producing a superior synthesis of thought and forms of life. According to Engels (1925), the universe, in its entirety, works dialectically.

Engels' position, from which Vygotsky draws inspiration, is clearly distant from a mechanic and physicalist vision of the world of ideas and reality, and it involves, methodologically, any kind of cognitive enterprise. Nevertheless, in the cultural and scientific debate that surfaced after the October Revolution, the mechanist direction broadly spread. Probably, this was due to a general limited philosophical criterion, and the "mechanic" perspective was perceived, generally, as more materialistic than the "dialectic" one.

It is not a case that after Lenin's death, those sectors of Soviet science that were more detached, in their essence, from the dialectic perspective of the theory of knowledge and more linked to a mechanist vision of the world showed a negative attitude towards psychoanalysis and the scientific discoveries taking place in the West, in those years. In the field of physics, the works by Einstein, Planck, and Bohr were generally criticised. The general reductionist instance was applied to the relation between science and common sense and, viewing the qualitative differences between superior and inferior forms of knowledge as null, distrust manifested towards any scientific theory that deviated too neatly from those features of intuitiveness and evidence that characterised our daily thinking. For those who belonged to this cluster, psychoanalysis was, of course, something to be contrasted. The philosopher Varjas (1925), representative of the "mechanist" approach, was one of those thinkers who – even though not in a systematic way – held this attitude towards Freudian ideas.

Without delving too deeply into a comparison between "mechanist" and "dialectic", we should note that both Vygotsky and Eisenstein assumed the dialectical perspective in the methodological dimension of their work. On a more political level, the debate pro or against mechanistic reductionism raised the question of the possibility of bringing back, or even reducing, the area of psychology and, in general, of human disciplines to a material level of development of productive forces.

It was Lenin who defended the so-called "bourgeois specialists" that other figures of the revolutionary movement like Bogdanov and Lunacharsky, members of Proletkult, wanted to sideline. A faction of the Bolsheviks harboured the dream to give life to radically new science and culture. An alleged incompatibility was advanced between the necessity of the revolutionary movement to develop its own autonomy in the domain of culture and scientific and cultural achievements that had grown before the revolution. In practice, this materialised into a general hostility towards any collaboration with representative figures of pre-revolutionary culture and science. Lenin, on the other hand, believed that theories of different levels could contradict each other without denying the fact that new theories could deepen or contradict previous theories. The idea of creating a totally proletarian science and culture looked to the most important figure of the revolution, a chimeric waste of energy.

This would have increased the risk of underestimating the historically gained scientific and cultural elements. It was necessary to face the impellent problem of the transformation of a semi-illiterate country into a working democracy. The attitude of Lenin towards Ivan Pavlov was exemplary. In fact, it was thanks to Lenin that Pavlov could develop his works and enjoy an effective experimental situation. Moreover, thanks to the support of the Soviet leader, in April 1918, a few months before the revolution, an agreement with the Academy of Sciences was signed that allowed autonomy and freedom of research for scientists. Lenin did not share the illusion that the cultural revolution could transform every Soviet citizen into a scientist, abolishing any distinction between specialists and non-specialists. In fact, he feared that such an idea could lead to an inappropriate expansion of the diffusive and popular aspects of culture, to the detriment of critical and creative ones, essential to the creation of the new socialist society.

The characteristics of Pavlov's objective and experimental research corresponded to methodological criteria, which were opposite, on a philosophical level, to the metaphysical approach. That is the reason Lenin appreciated Pavlov's ideas. Lenin's general attitude towards these assumptions is expressed in one of his notes on the use of metaphysics in psychology:

> This is a most obvious symptom of metaphysics, with which every science began: as long as people did not know how to set about studying the facts, they always invented *a priori* general theories, which were always sterile. The metaphysician-chemist, still unable to make a factual investigation of chemical processes, concocts a theory about chemical affinity as a force. The metaphysician-biologist talks about the nature of life and vital force. The metaphysician-psychologist argues about the nature of the soul. Here is the

> method itself that is absurd. You cannot argue about the soul without having explained psychical processes in particular: here progress must consist precisely in abandoning general theories and philosophical discourses about the nature of the soul, and in being able to put the study of the facts about particular psychical processes on a scientific footing ... The scientific psychologist has discarded philosophical theories on *the* soul and set about making a direct study of the material substrate of psychical phenomena – the nervous processes.
>
> *(Lenin, 1894; Engl. transl., p. 144)*

As a matter of fact, this statement is quite inconsistent in relation to the general dialectical and materialistic thought of the October Revolution leader. It is a mechanistic conception that, if endorsed by the Soviet psychologists of his time, would have relegated psychology to the enclosure of physiology.

Vygotsky certainly agreed with a materialistic notion of the psyche and made a different theoretical proposal according to which the material basis of human consciousness is not to be searched in the neural system – that, of course, exists and belongs to human beings – but in the historical and cultural dimension, in the environmental and temporal context in which human psyche develops.

Therefore, as a material basis of the psyche, it is correct to think of historical reality, rather than matter, in the Cartesian way, as an extension of space. History is real even if we cannot touch it (with a finger). Therefore, in Vygotsky's cultural and historical perspective, it is correct to make the hypothesis of a realistic notion of psyche, conscious and unconscious.

In its turn, even if philosophically lacking with respect to the dialectical aspects of the psyche and the world, Pavlovism prevailed within Soviet psychology for its homogeneity with the entire tradition of Materialism, even if mechanist. This advantage of Pavlov's theory allowed it to thrive even after the resolution of the Central Committee of the Communist Party on the fourth of July 1936. This resolution, related to the "pedological distortions" (see the text in Caroli and Mecacci, 2020) and based on an abstract interpretation of Marxist principles, ended up crystallising the entire picture of Soviet psychology for decades.

Many original research perspectives dissolved, including the cultural-historical theory of Vygotsky. Psychoanalysis was not directly affected; in fact, since the late 1920s, the psychoanalytical debate, under the political pressure of the regime's theorists, had gradually died out. Vygotsky continued to express interest in psychoanalysis in his work *Pedagogical Psychology* (1926) and *Lectures on Psychology* (1932b). By the early 1930s, the Russian Psychoanalytic Society came to an end, and many supporters of psychoanalysis returned to their hometowns.

Some aspects of the human and intellectual difficulties Vygotsky faced were like those encountered by Eisenstein. They were both Jewish and came from bourgeois families. After the revolution, anti-Semitism was still present in Russia, and both could be accused of proximity to Trotsky's ideas. Additionally, they both had been close to people criticised for their ideologies or even labelled as "enemies of the people". Vygotsky was a friend of Mandelstam, and Eisenstein was a friend of Mayakovsky. Forced to hard labour, Mandelstam died in a gulag in 1938 as a result of Stalin's actions of purging the country, while Mayakovski, due to personal emotional issues and to the campaign against him led by the party, committed suicide. Both Vygotsky and Eisenstein had taken an interest in psychoanalysis. They supported psychoanalytical ideas, and by the early 1930s, in the years of the Stalinist "Great Terror", this was a sufficient reason to be arrested and convicted. This happened to many intellectuals of the time (see Conquest, 1973).

Lenin never took a position towards psychoanalysis, but the context of his ideas showed there were no contact points between his ideas and psychoanalytical thought, and he generally held a negative theoretical attitude towards psychoanalysis. Tögel (1989) stated that both Lenin and his wife Krupskaya were aware of psychoanalytical theories. Tögel found some Russian translations of Freud in Lenin's personal library, with handwritten notes by Krupskaya. Moreover, as Tögel recalls, one of the greatest Russian neuropathologists, Livery Darkshevich (1858–1925), one of Lenin's personal physicians, had been a friend of Freud's when he was young. After Lenin's death, Clara Zetkin published his memoirs in Russian, and she claimed that he had made the following statements about "a pamphlet on the sex questions written by a Communist authoress" where a reference to Freud was given:

> The mention of Freud's hypotheses is designed to give the pamphlet a scientific veneer, but it is so bungling by an amateur. Freud's theory has now become a fad. I mistrust sex theories expounded in articles, treatises, pamphlets, etc. – in short, the theories dealt with in that specific literature which sprouts so luxuriantly on the dung heap of bourgeois society. I mistrust those who are always absorbed in the sex problems, the way an Indian saint is absorbed in the contemplation of his navel. It seems to me that this superabundance of sex theories, which for the most part are mere hypotheses, and often quite arbitrary ones, stems from a personal need. It springs from the desire to justify one's own abnormal or excessive sex life before bourgeois morality and to plead for tolerance towards oneself. This veiled respect for bourgeois morality is as repugnant to me as rooting about in all that bears on sex. No matter how rebellious and revolutionary it may be made to appear, it is in the final analysis thoroughly bourgeois. Intellectuals and others like them are *particularly* keen on this. There is no room for it in the Party, among the class-conscious, fighting proletariat.
>
> *(Zetkin, 1925; Engl. transl., p. 101)*

Pravda reported these notes with promptness and claimed that Lenin himself opposed the attempt to outline points of contact between Marxism and psychoanalysis. Petrovskij (1967, p. 116) marked 1925 as the year in which a large-scale attack against psychoanalysis started.

It is plausible that Lenin's criticism was governed not only by his opposition to Freudian theories but also by the many problems related to the new ideal and moral ideas that revolutionary change had evoked. Among these problems, it was not only sexual life but also the relationship between man and woman and communist ethics to be the object of political and theoretical attention. Some articles in the form of *Letters to the Working Youth* were written by the communist leader Aleksandra Kollontai (1922, 1923a, 1923b) and drew much attention. Regardless of the historical reasons for this issue, it must be remembered that the debate significantly involved Soviet intellectuals. Unluckily, Kollontai received many protests in response to the *Letters*, and even if she distanced herself from any consumerist and physiological conception of sex, her name became polemically related to sexually permissive and lax behaviours.

Lenin was always extremely polemical towards sexual theories that did not involve the individual's personality and sociality, and he criticised Kollontai's ideas on the grounds of their detachment from historical objectivity and the exasperation on the individual dimension (see Angelini, 1988, p. 155).

From a wider perspective, it should be noted that within the multi-layered context of the lively Soviet cultural world, psychoanalytical thought spread and was nourished by the debate. At the same time and in relation to the same topic, however, psychoanalysis had been subjected to sharp criticism.

The journal *Pod Znamenem Marksisma*, founded in 1922, hosted a lively debate on psychoanalysis where controversial opinions emerged. The journal also published the writings of several theorists, already mentioned, who conformed to the regime's cultural policy. By virtue of this discriminating criterion, they attacked psychoanalysis and any proposal, such as that of Vygotsky, that appeared dissimilar to theirs.

Worth of mention are the works of Abram M. Deborin (1928), Vladimir A. Iurinets (1925), and Isay D. Sapir (1929–1930) (see Angelini, 1988, Chapters 9 and 11). Moreover, in the volume *Freudianism* (1927), Valentin N. Voloshinov – while attributing a certain therapeutic validity to psychoanalysis – minutely contested the theoretical hypotheses expressed, in support of psychoanalysis, in the well-known work *Psychology and Marxism* (1925), edited by Kornilov.

Moreover, authoritative sources[1] attribute the above-mentioned work to Michail Bakhtin (1895–1975), one of the most important Russian theorists of literary studies. Psychoanalysis was accused of being a "world conception", and its scientific validity was opposed. The great theoretical and methodological contributions of psychoanalytical thought were being removed from the pressures of politics and the constraints of ideology that were increasingly dominant within the regime.

Note

1 See Ponzio, *Introduction* to Voloshinov (1927; Ital. transl., p. 7).

4

EISENSTEIN AND PSYCHOANALYSIS

Eisenstein was deeply interested in psychoanalysis, even though he had some contradictions. On a chronological level, references to Freud in *Memoirs* are quite early. Eisenstein recalls his first enthusiastic reading of *Leonardo da Vinci and a Memory of His Childhood* (Eisenstein, 1997; Ital. transl., 2006, p. 242), which gave him the opportunity to interpret his own creative energy in terms of sublimation. In his life, he neared psychoanalytical ideas from an intellectual point of view, and he met several representative figures of the first generation of psychoanalysis. Eisenstein recalls having read, after his first approach with Freud, *Die Bedeutung der Psychoanalyse für die Geisteswissenschaften* (*Psychoanalysis and its Applications*, 1913) by Hans Sachs and Otto Rank. Rice (see Rice, 1993, pp. 121, 123) claims that these authors delved into Russian literature and, in particular, into the psychoanalytical dimension of Dostoevsky, even before Freud dedicated his thoughts to the author (Freud, 1928); this is a further element to understand the director's interest towards both of them. Eisenstein, recalling with affection Sachs, wrote:

> I actually met Hans Sachs, - that marvellous, bespectacled, wise old salamander and his terrifying African mask - a 'symbol of complexes' which hung above his small low patients' couch, in Berlin many years later. We became great friends. He gave me a most interesting book about psychoanalysis, *Versuch einer Genitaltheorie* [Essay in genital theory], by Ferenczi, which explained a great deal of things (admittedly *post factum*!) which I had come across on my obsessive quest to penetrate the secrets of ecstasy.
>
> *(Eisenstein, 1995, p. 600)*

Eisenstein was particularly attracted to the works of Otto Rank and Sandor Ferenczi for their interest in archaic mental states.

DOI: 10.4324/9781003398554-5

Moreover, this focus on the origin and history of psychological development crosses all the director's intellectual production. On the other hand, his relations with psychoanalysis showed some contradictions.

Eisenstein's Marxist culture, oriented towards praxis and spontaneous inclination, as an artist with an inclination towards "doing", made it difficult for him, in specific circumstances, to address a discipline focused on the subject and – at that time – still paying little attention to the dimension of collective social history. He also wrote, referring to Freud: "The curse of knowledge that could not liberate him overlies all psychoanalysis" (Eisenstein, 1995, p. 355).

Nonetheless, Eisenstein supported psychoanalytical ideas. However, one should remember that in the second part of his life, as happened to many other Soviet intellectuals who had lived through the October Revolution, he could no longer express these ideas.

In *Rezhissura: Iskusstvo mizanstseny* (*Direction: The Art of Staging*), written between 1932 and 1933 for the students of the Muscovite State Institute of Cinematography, where he taught Direction, there is a critical note on psychoanalysis (Eisenstein, 1932–1933; Ital. transl., pp. 586–592). At that time, amid the Stalinist reaction, psychoanalysis was under attack from the regime's fundamentalist theorists, and the Moscow Psychoanalytic Society had to be disbanded due to the opposing political climate.

At the time, Eisenstein expressed doubts about the capability of psychoanalytical theory to interpret the dynamics of artistic creativity fully. Nevertheless, on the same pages, he could not help but write:

> It is undeniable that the results of psychoanalysis are especially useful to navigate the territory of neuropsychiatry. For pathological cases, the Freudian scheme corresponds in many ways to the actual order of things.
>
> *(Eisenstein, 1932–1933; see Ital. transl., p. 587)*

At that stage, Freud's name had already been deleted from specialised journals and the press (Angelini, 1988, p. 177). It was not possible to name him, not even to criticise his ideas, but Eisenstein's literary and essay production testifies to the influence of Freudian ideas, even at that time.

By virtue of his good relationship with Sachs, he invited Eisenstein, in October 1929, to speak at a conference at the Psychoanalytic Institute of Berlin, the most important centre for research and education in the field of psychoanalysis, between the two wars. Eisenstein gave his speech on *Wichmannstrasse* 10 at the Institute headquarters, whose interior had been renovated and furnished by the architect Ernst Freud, son of Sigmund Freud.

On this occasion, the director spoke of the conflicting nature of the expressive movement in terms of a contrast between unconscious drives and the will that aims to restrain and refrain them.

The Institute's archive has disappeared, so we do not precisely know the reactions to Eisenstein's speech, but the event had an impact. Kurt Lewin was among the audience, and unlike many of his academic colleagues, he was particularly interested in psychoanalysis. He believed that film could be used as a research tool in the field of psychology.

At the time, Lewin – who later became a well-known supporter of Gestalt psychology – often met Ernst Cassirer and Wolfgang Köhler, one of the most important Gestalt thinkers in academic circles. Lewin took an interest in the director. He had been introduced to Eisenstein's work by Aleksandr Luria through a letter representing a sort of long-distance introduction and presentation.

Shortly afterwards, on the third of December 1929, Lewin wrote to the director, who was in London at the time:

> Dear Eisenstein, I have thought a lot about your speech. I want you to know that your theory on expressive movement is more important to me than the writings of all the psychologists of today. I have already spoken to Köhler, and he will send you an invitation so we will be able to discuss the various possibilities as soon as you are here.
>
> *(Bulgakowa, 2001, footnote 11, p. 182)*

Soon after, Eisenstein received a letter from Wolfgang Köhler, the director of the Institute of Psychology:

> Dear Sir, my colleague Kurt Lewin informed me of your research in the field of psychological issues *related* to expression and told me you have achieved very important results and formulated very important observations in this field, that have drawn my attention.
>
> *(Bulgakowa, 2001, footnote 9, p. 182)*

Due to overlapping appointments, Eisenstein could not speak at the Institute, but Köhler's letter is important. Even though, at that time, the Berlin Academy had rejected psychoanalysis, Eisenstein's proposals and his activities attracted attention.

Kurt Lewin had started making short documentaries as early as 1923, mostly to record expressions, emotions, and movements in children. According to his assistant Bluma Wulfovna Zeigarnik, who would later become an important psychologist in the Soviet world, with those films, Lewin laid the foundations for the development of his "Field Theory".

As we know, according to this theory, personality and its environment must be considered as a single constellation. The aspiration to grasp psychological phenomena according to interacting and complex structures is inherent in Lewin's ideas. It is possible that Eisenstein, a supporter of a dialectical vision of phenomena, viewed this position with approval. According to Bulgakova (1989, p. 89), the director's dialectical perspective proposed the dynamic concepts of sequence and structure, going far beyond the simplified notion of an antagonistic pair.

Zeigarnik stated that Eisenstein participated in several shooting days of films directed by Lewin. The director then had a chance to see most of Lewin's film documentation (see Bulgakova, 1989, p. 82).

Informed by Eisenstein, Luria organised a research group on film psychology in the late 1920s with the participation of Vygotsky, Marr, and Eisenstein himself. A laboratory was created at the Institute of Cinematography to realise various typologies of filming for scientific purposes.

According to Bulgakowa (2001, p. 178 ff.), the participation of Eisenstein in the Berlin Psychoanalytic Conference is historically important because, on this occasion, the director shed light on his detachment from intellectual cinema and from the mechanistic positions of Pavlovism to underline his interest in psychoanalysis and get closer to the Gestalt approach. After his return to the Soviet Union, there would be no more opportunities to speak officially and openly on psychoanalysis or other Western psychological theories.

As previously mentioned, in the 1930s and 1940s, the ideological climate was hostile to Freud in the USSR; any reference to psychoanalysis in works intended for publication had to be removed or encrypted.

Luckily, before the October Revolution, many texts of psychoanalysis had been translated and published in Russia. The *Three Essays on the Theory of Sexuality* (1905) by Freud and *The Content of the Psychoses* (1908) by Jung had both been translated into Russian in 1909. Since then, while Jung's work had been neglected – except for a partial version of *Psychological Types* (1921), in 1924, almost all of Freud's multi-decade production had been translated.[1] The last work to be translated in Russia was *The Future of an Illusion* (1927) in 1928. In the first two decades of the twentieth century, before the affirmation of the dogmatic and mechanist ideology promoted by Stalinism, Russia had elaborated its own strand of thought and achieved an autonomous presence within the international psychoanalytical movement.

It is in this context that Eisenstein's ideas on psychoanalysis and the theoretical heritage of Marxism must be evaluated. The framework of the director's thought is connected to Marxist dialectic. From a theoretical point of view, he elaborated a connection, or rather an authentically dialectical relationship, between consciousness and instinct. According to Eisenstein, the basic taxonomic schemes that assess the superiority of one pole over the other must be overcome. On this basis, also in a psychoanalytical sense, the regression towards the lowest levels of consciousness, to which the director gave a theoretical centrality, finds in art one of its privileged expressions. He sees the artistic process as a pattern of liberation and expression of the deep, regressed contents of the psyche.

This position, which rejects the idea of a dominating immersion, operated by "stronger" areas of the mind at the expense of "weaker" ones, in a Soviet social scenario, had conceptual analogies of political nature. It echoed the image of a communist society with no rigid and mechanical division between the *revolutionary* avant-garde and the *masses*. Added to this, there was the reverie of a world without social classes where the past would be overcome, but not denied, a past capable of supporting the value of primitive, non-differentiated thinking against the individuality and singularity of the modern capitalist world. In the words of Etkin:

> He often likened ecstatic, undifferentiated states of consciousness (the "pre-psyche") to the classless society. For him, the proto-psyche offered a psychological ideal, much as Engels saw his social ideals in the classless, promiscuous social grouping. In such primitive ideas, the past and the future, progress and regress are confounded, just as male and female, subject and object, individual *and* mass are commingled. Nonetheless, a perfect commingling proved unattainable.
> *(Etkind, 1997, p. 320)*

This was a theoretical possibility within the philosophical debate on Marxist thought. Conceptually, it went far beyond the debate on art and aesthetics and made it difficult for him to deal with the Stalinist theoretical apparatus.

In these ideas, we see some notions that belonged to a mature Eisenstein, and that became apparent, above all, in the later years of his life, in particular, the theme of "prenatal" or "intrauterine" memory, significantly influenced by psychoanalytical concepts. Eisenstein believed that this type of memory, formed in a "pre-individual life", could play a key role at the unconscious level. These hypotheses are expressed in various sections of *Metod* and his *Memoirs*, written in 1946.

In many of his works, Eisenstein speculated on the issue of regression in terms of a process capable of going backwards to primordial forms of life and existence. Eisenstein referred to single-celled organisms and the foetus in a mother's womb. He referred to the desire for a return to the mother – which he had begun investigating, theoretically, in the early 1930s till the end of his life – with the German expression *Mutterleibversenkung* (*sinking into the womb*). The term was often shortened in the acronym MLB, taken probably from Franz Alexander's article *Der biologische Sinn psychischer Vorgänge (über Buddhas Versenkungslehre)* [*The Biological Sense of Psychological Processes (on Buddha's Theory of Immersion)*] (1923). It represents a further hint at the influence of Freudian theories on the director's ideas.

Eisenstein dealt with these themes particularly in the essay dedicated to Walt Disney and in some parts of *Metod* and the *Memoirs*. He shed light on various aspects of the foetus' intrauterine life, leaving a mark on the history of the arts. The aim was to elaborate, artistically, the topic of regression in the womb. Conceptually, Eisenstein began to be interested in intrauterine life (see *Memoirs*, 2006, p. 448) when he was trying to interpret a broad framework related to anthropological, ethnological, and mass psychology phenomena. The director wanted to explore the issue of ecstasy in which he was extremely interested, often referred to as a sort of "sinking in".

This subject, more than any other, promoted the director's encounter with psychoanalytical ideas in harmony with the work by Franz Alexander (1923). According to Bordwell (1993, p. 194), in the concept of ecstasy, Eisenstein also welcomed Wilhelm Reich's suggestions on sexuality. The director was aware of Reich's work since he had contacts with the Berlin Psychoanalytic Society. Reich had many ordeals in the USSR and got in touch with the Soviet political world.

In 1929, Reich spent two months in the Soviet Union, staying in Moscow, where he lectured at the Communist Academy (see Etkind, 1993, pp. 294–296). As one can imagine, he was unable to persuade the members of the Academy on the necessity of sexual revolution, "Later he would accuse "those scoundrels" in Moscow of organising a campaign against him in the German Communist Party" (Etkind, 1997, p. 243). Shortly after, in 1930, Reich moved from Wien to Berlin. The move came at the end of a painful and fraught period, of which we find indirect historical evidence in some letters Freud wrote to his impetuous pupil (Angelini, 2013). Even in the German capital, Reich's intellectual recklessness was not welcomed. Within a year, between 1933 and 1934, he was expelled from both the International Psychoanalytic Association and the German Communist Party.

His fellow psychoanalysts saw him as a dangerous political extremist, while his fellow party members thought he was a corrupt bourgeois because he raised the issue of sexuality. Reich and Eisenstein had read each other's work,[2] and in 1934, the director asked the psychologist to send him a copy of *The Function of the Orgasm* (1927), which could be used for his analysis of ecstasy (see Bulgakowa, 2001, p. 172).

Eisenstein's ideas on ecstasy are conceptually much broader than the sexual dimension advocated by Reich. Eisenstein's main inspiration, with respect to the notion of ecstasy, came mostly from the ideas of Otto Rank and Sandor Ferenczi. They both gave centrality to the concept of trauma and its psychological foundational value. In the same year, 1924, Ferenczi published *Thalassa. Essay on the Theory of Genitality* and Rank published *The Trauma of Birth and its Psychoanalytical Meaning*.

In these works, Eisenstein looked for ideas to elaborate his idea of a regress back to the original, following a line that, in a regressive sense, aimed to elevate the value of artwork.

At the time, he had probably already read *The Significance of Psychoanalysis for the Human Sciences* (1913), written by Otto Rank and Hanns Sachs and *The Incest Theme in Literature and Legend* (1912) by Rank. Rank's ideas diverged from Freud's, and he was criticised by the latter.

While Freud, in his first theoretical proposals, stated that anxiety came from unconscious neurotic conflicts that affect the area of sexuality, Rank associated anxiety with the distressing experience of birth. At the same time, Rank believed that every experience of pleasure tended to replicate the original pleasure of being in the womb. The biological trauma of birth, which is to say, the loss of that original pleasure, had a crucial role in the psyche.

This idea is in contrast with Freud's, who investigated the unconscious on a specifically psychological level, whereas Rank investigated unconscious phenomena, placing their origin in a somatic trauma. According to Rank, the deepest biological strata are linked, unconsciously, to the highest conscious contents of mental production, as if high and low could correspond to each other.

Moreover, Rank developed the idea of an unconscious and continuous desire to return to the mother's womb and this longing found expression in sexual satisfaction and various forms of religious sublimation and artistic idealisation.

Rank identified the trauma of the child's separation from its mother with the first experience of anxiety, the so-called "proto anxiety". The child reacts to the trauma, organising its psychological life through ghosts and forming its own identity, although the desire to return to the mother's womb remains in the unconscious. Each episode of anxiety experienced in adulthood is related to the trauma of birth.

Even if Eisenstein found inspiration in Rank's ideas, the director's ideas did not overlap with Rank's. As Lena Corritore stated,

> If Rank claims the existence of an unconscious, incessantly renewed desire to return to the mother's womb, which finds expressions in sexual satisfaction and in various forms of religious sublimation and artistic idealisation, Eisenstein seeks the expressions of this drive in the material and compositional structure of artworks from any time and any place.
>
> *(see Lena Corritore, 2021a, in press)*

Eisenstein questions the *Grundproblem*, the *fundamental question* of the laws that govern the creation of a work of art. In line with Marxist orientation, according to Eisenstein, these laws were those of dialectic, and they were universal; they simultaneously controlled the development of nature and man, even in its social dimension. Within this perspective, Eisenstein was inclined to think that the unconscious corresponded to a stage of primordial development of the psyche, characterised by a form of sensory thought related to archaic biological phenomena.

With concern for the nature of these phenomena, Eisenstein was interested in the period prior to the presence of the individual in the world. It is a period that begins with conception, continues through the prenatal phase, and ends with birth:

> The interest in the prenatal phase has always been very strong for me and this interest soon extended to the existence that preceded the species. I became interested in the phases of biological development, the stages preceding the human stage! Going even further, my interest extended to the earliest forms of social relations: the primitive society before the division in social classes, the specific forms of behaviour and thought. And all these issues have drawn my interest

> as a form of permanence of all those stages within our consciousness, in our thought and behaviour.
>
> *(Eisenstein, 2006; Ital. transl., pp. 358, 359)*

In fact, Eisenstein went even further compared to Rank and put forward the hypothesis that individuals retain the memory of the moment of their conception, of the *amphimixis*, the fusion of the *nuclei* (*pronuclei*) of the gametes, or sex cells (egg and sperm) that are combined in the act of conception. According to the director, this is the primitive experience of ecstasy. It is precisely ecstasy (coming out of oneself) that Eisenstein aims to evoke with his art in the spectators;

> *Pathos* is what forces the spectators to jump while sitting in their seats. It is pathos that forces them to snap, to clap, to shout. It is what makes their eyes shine with enthusiasm before tears of excitement roll down their cheeks. In other words, it is everything that drives the spectators *out of themselves*.
>
> *(Eisenstein, 2006; Ital. transl., p. 368)*

Even in this artistic enterprise conducted for the benefit of the viewer, the philosophical categories of Marxism and, specifically, of dialectical materialism remain as a backdrop and offer a universal method useful at every level of investigation (see Aumont, 1979). The ecstasy of *amphimixis*, outlined by Eisenstein, who drew inspiration from Rank's ideas, is conceived as a dialectical moment of the passage from quantity to quality and the realisation of the unity of opposites.

Eisenstein expanded his ideas also through the influence of Ferenczi. Differently from Rank, who denied the possibility of real reminiscences related to the moment of conception, locating the origin of mnestic activity in the act of birth or in the foetal period, Ferenczi, in his ontogenetic and phylogenetic theory of genitality, put forward the hypothesis of a regressive activity of the unconscious, which was not limited to pre-human periods on the evolutionary scale… and admitted the possibility of unconscious mnestic residues related to the moment of division of matter into "organic and inorganic" (Lena Corritore, 2021b, in press).

The experience of ecstasy is central to Eisenstein, and this experience, promoted by the force of art pathos, echoes the "zero point" of conception. Therefore, his goal is to create works whose artistic qualities recall, in the unconscious, nostalgia for the ecstatic intrauterine fulfilment. In the director's perspective, this moment of artistic fruition even goes so far as to have political consequences.

As Lena Corritore stated, "it meant to act on the spectators' consciousness in a subliminal way, inducing them first to desire the return (reactionary nostalgia) and then the future advent (progressive ideal) of a social structure without social class division" (Lena Corritore, 2021b, in press).

Based on these foundations, Eisenstein defines art as "organic" since it functions by means of the same laws that govern natural phenomena:

> In an organic artwork, the elements that make up the whole also participate in each individual component. The same law runs through the whole and each of its parts, but also through different planes against which the whole is created. Independently from the planes, they contain the same principles which manifest each time in a specific way. Given this condition, it is possible to speak of the organic nature of a work of art, provided one conceives the concept of *organism* in the way Engels defines it in the *Dialectic of Nature*: "The 'organism' is *certainly* the superior unity" ... The organicity and the feeling of organicity produced by the work of art arise when the law of creation of artwork corresponds to the *laws of structuring the phenomena of nature*. ... We are faced, in this case, with a work of art – an *artificial work of art* – created with the same laws that give structure to *non*-artificial phenomena – the *organic* phenomena of nature.
>
> *(Eisenstein, 1981; Ital. transl., pp. 14, 15)*

In this way, the work of art can also be "effective" because it exerts power over emotions.

As previously mentioned, Eisenstein was also influenced by Sandor Ferenczi, another important psychoanalytical author who was one of Freud's favourite learners. Attracted by the possibilities of regression towards primitive thought, Eisenstein was significantly impressed by Ferenczi's *Versuch einer Genitaltheorie* (1924), later known as *Thalassa*.

Ferenczi considered the sexual act central to his "Theory of Genitality"; he considered it as an attempt to re-establish the lost unity with the maternal body. This unity was regained, momentarily, in coitus. He also passionately believed that there was a significant parallelism between ontogeny and phylogeny. He claimed that the infant's detachment from the "aquatic" nature of intrauterine life was a reiteration, at each birth, of the process of adaptation of mammals to terrestrial life after the drying up of the sea in the past.

In his ontogenetic and phylogenetic theory of genitality, Ferenczi put forward the hypothesis of the existence of a trace of unconscious psychism dating back to the moment of the separation of organic from inorganic matter. Like Freud, he appreciated Lamarck's ideas on evolutionism and interpreted coitus not only as a hallucinatory and symbolic attempt to re-establish the intrauterine situation by escaping the trauma of birth but also phylogenetically, like a "thalassic regression", a desire to return to the ocean abandoned in the past by the aquatic vertebrates, ancestors of mankind.

His ideas were quite different from Rank's traumatic description of birth. At the end of his essay, Ferenczi highlighted a parallelism between the desire for a return to the maternal womb and the instinct of death outlined a few years earlier by Freud (1920), which had a profound impact on Eisenstein.

As Lena Corritore stated:

> This is the original situation ("the first spark"), a model of the law of dialectic movement and symbol of his idea of art and filmmaking, that the director synthetises in the collection of drawings called *EX-STASIS* (Nuevo Laredo, 1932) which became the basis of his "operative aesthetics" ... The director often refers to MLB in his theoretical observations, investigating the possible aspects: both when he analyses foetal existence traces within the history of art and when, referring to the "fundamental biogenetic law" by Haeckel, looks at aspects which are more directly related to primitive stages of evolution of living species.
>
> *(Lena Corritore, 2021b, in press)*

According to Eisenstein, the main task of the artist (*Grundproblem*), on the aesthetical level, was to re-activate, through artworks, these regressive feelings, making them capable of producing an emotional involvement. The idea of "sinking in the maternal womb", discussed from several viewpoints by psychoanalytical authors, was considered, on an artistic level, the most interesting and productive form of regression. On several occasions, Eisenstein expressed the idea that the "sinking" into ecstasy described by mystics was the feeling of going back, "sinking into" the maternal womb.

In his *Memoirs*, in *Monsieur, Madame et Bébé* he says:

> Much has been written on the return to the maternal womb (e.g., Doctor Alexander on nirvana in "Imago"). On "being born" Rank wonderfully wrote in *Das Trauma der Geburt*... Ferenczi expressed his ideas on these topics in *Versuch einer Genitaltheorie* adding the issue regarding the drive towards death. And even regress through "forms" of animated nature to ... the unanimated stage!
>
> *(Eisenstein, 2006; Ital. transl., pp. 370, 371)*

He wrote that, by reading Ferenczi, he made

> the acquaintance of our most common ancestor at the lowest level of the transition from plant to animal world. From its fish-line form, *science* considers it the official progenitor even of that first level from which the exciting variety of evolution began, as Darwin perceived.
>
> *(Eisenstein, 2006; Ital. transl., p. 448)*

As far as the connection with Marxist thought is concerned, the topic of biological evolutionism, in a philosophical evaluation, is extensively discussed by Engels (1925). Engels agrees with the Hegelian critique of empiricism, which was blamed for its disregard of all theories, as well as for its unequivocal consideration of "facts" only considered as reliable and indisputable unquestionable data.

The effort to adhere rigidly only to the observed facts, without fuelling theory, could paradoxically inhibit the innovative force of Darwinism. Behind these positions lay controversial evaluations of the use of the philosophical tools of induction and deduction, which cannot be explored in depth here (see Cervini, 2010, p. 69). Engels also claimed, with respect to Darwinian theory, the indispensable intertwining of chance and necessity in both scientific and historical issues. By introducing the concept of chance to explain the possible modifications of the species, Darwinism freed itself from all teleological constraints. In fact, teleology demanded the notion of necessity.

Eliminating the notion of necessity from the theory of evolution erased any dialectical perspective to favour a mechanistic theoretical scenario. Engels wrote:

> For example, the development of a concept or of a conceptual relation (positive and negative, cause and effect, substance and essence) in the history of thought, is in relation to its development in the mind of the individual dialectician like the development of an organism in palaeontology is in relation to its development in embryology (or rather in history and in the individual embryo). This was first demonstrated by Hegel with concern to concepts. In historical development, causality plays a role that is *included in necessity* both in dialectical thought and in the development of the embryo.
>
> *(Engels, 1925, p. 232)*

Engels and the Soviet intellectuals who supported him believed that Darwinian theory could confirm its validity "only as the practical proof of Hegel's account of the inner connection between necessity and chance" (Engels, 1925; Engl. transl., p. 229). The preservation of dialectical philosophy was at stake. Engels was looking for a single law of development, which would not crystallise in a single explanatory instance but in the dialectical confrontation between opposing principles, whereby the latter is the negation of the former and the reunion of the two is the superior and organic synthesis.

On a historical level, this translated into the attempt to identify a multifaceted scheme in which different and opposing principles intertwine, provide an explanation for the multiform unity that is human history. Engels criticised Darwin's idea of the struggle for survival of the fittest and the species; he considered it little articulated and insufficient to cope with the complexity of human historical processes. Two were the elements that, according to him, had to come together in the concept of evolution: *progress* and *regress*. This was the starting point to identify the *fundamental law* of nature and history, which lay in both simultaneously.

In the last section of the chapter entitled *Still on Expressive Movement* (in the work *On Biomechanics*, 2009) – written between 1922 and 1940 – Eisenstein embraced the Engelsian concepts afore illustrated. As Cervini stated, he outlined the research of

> diverse theoretical framework, in which the phenomena of consciousness, creative processes and works of art (products of the creative process), were

> supposed to represent the result of an interpenetration of opposing forces and tendencies, converging into a supreme and more complex unity. This unity cannot reveal the supremacy of one principle over another, of one tendency over another, but it mirrors the reciprocal passage and interaction of forces aimed to the construction of a new harmony. This idea, just as with Engels, had an immediate historical-political resonance.
>
> *(Cervini, 2010, pp. 71, 72)*

In other words, the director opposed the idea of a *hierarchy of contents*, both in the social and psychological context. A hierarchy would be opposed to a universally dialectical vision of the world. In the words of Eisenstein:

> In my field of action I would never allow the idea of interpenetration among "superior or inferior" levels, or pulling and braking, *avant-gardist* or *backward*, and this is the same idea expressed by comrade Stalin – in another disciplinary domain – in relation to *the remains of past in consciousness*. I would like to associate this issue of the relation among different levels to the way Engels outlined this interpenetration which exists in nature … We live in a society in which the principle of war based on all against all has been overcome, a society in which the basic principle of the struggle for survival has been erased, as well as the supremacy of one class over another, of one nation over another, a society in which our consciousness, reflecting this unusual order of things … cannot but introduce a new perspective of harmony, collaboration, and interaction; that is to say the convergency of a supreme unity of all these principles, perceived as opposing poles connected as a whole, inevitably trespassing their borders, interacting in order to achieve a unity of form and content. This process manifests both in the concept of method and practice. Not only in method, but also in style.
>
> *(Eisenstein, 2009; Ital. transl., pp. 113–115)*

In the last part of the above chapter, Eisenstein also put forward political and "class" motivations, but his proposal is universal and leads to the opening of an authentically historical space based on man as a species. Hence his interest in Lévy-Bruhl's work, from which he draws the idea of a *pre-logical thought* enacted in the work of art, which explains the regression to the lowest strata of consciousness.

As the principle of explication of human thought, logic is relativised. Eisenstein is attracted to those experiences capable of highlighting the existence of states of consciousness and knowledge which are not controlled by generally rational criteria. This resulted in his interest, in the perspective outlined by his friend Vygotsky, in hypnotic states and dementia, religious and artistic ecstasy, and primitive or infantile thought. In illustrating his ideas, however, Eisenstein highlighted his detachment from any form of praise, direct or indirect, of irrationalism.

The director rejects the idea of a directional arrow, and he retains the idea of a model of the historical process that conjugates progress and regress and looks more like a spiral (universal growth scheme in organic phenomena) rather than a straight line directed towards an infinite and perfectible future.

In a general sense, Eisenstein's aim is the aesthetic question, delving into the *Grundproblem*, with the objective of understanding issues related to the evolution of the sensory organs. He outlines a *pre-logical* conception of artwork, which involves a sensual and emotional component, allowing the artistic product and, in particular, the cinematic product to approach forms of primitive thought.

In his own way, Eisenstein outlines a personal philosophy of history, wherein culture and expressive forms gain their meaning, expressed by human history. The enterprise, as outlined, is not limited to the anthropological and historical dimension, but it involves the biological reality and, in Engel's terms, the world as a whole. According to Eisenstein, in promoting this search, a very important figure was Luria. In the words of Eisenstein:

> My friend, consultant and usual advisor in all matters of this kind, Aleksandr Romanovich Luria, suggested me to read Goldschmidt's *Ascaris* which portrays, in a very poetic, comprehensible and scientifically thoughtful way, the fascinating picture of the vicissitudes of the formation of the *perfect* apparatuses of our organism from the earliest stages and levels of development.
>
> *(Eisenstein, 2006; Ital. transl., pp. 448, 449)*

Since the 1920s, the issue of regression had been nourished through contact with psychoanalysis and grew throughout Eisenstein's travels outside the Soviet Union.

In December 1930, Eisenstein went to Mexico, and from that moment, his theoretical and film production began to thrive in the "pre-logical" dimension, which fascinated him extensively. On his Mexican journey, he tangibly detected traces of cultures which were precedent to the colonial Catholic one, looking at that country's customs. Their rituals – from the practices of the community of *danzantes* to the flagellants of the processions in honour of the Virgin of Guadalupe – enact states of primitive ecstasy in the participants. In the chapter of *Metod* titled *Forward Momentum*, Mexico is described by Eisenstein as the "most ecstatic place of creation" (see Somaini, 2011, p. 262).

Mexico is the geographic and mental place where Eisenstein fantastically embraces free sensuality and the rediscovery of desires and drives in the regressive dive into the deepest layers of his own consciousness.

> What struck me most in my encounter with Mexico was the first sensation of that encounter: Mexico overturned everything we know about knowledge, consciousness, and the mirroring of reality in consciousness. I was struck, from the very first moment, by an extremely intense feeling, since the reality in front of me seemed generated by all the inclinations and passions that have always been living in me and still inhabit me.
>
> *(Eisenstein, 2020, vol. 1; Ital. transl., p. 234).*

Eisenstein's enthusiastic love for Mexico is rooted in strata that belong to history, anthropology and, simultaneously, psychology and art. The various levels connect simultaneously in a unified dimension. It is a co-presence that seems to echo the combination of different and redundant styles of Mexican buildings and monuments. The idea of death, in *Que viva Mexico!* (1931), which affirms the power of life in a carnivalesque way, is itself redeemed by the developmental capabilities of social forms created by the human being.

From these stimuli, during his journey to Mexico, Eisenstein started drawing again, modernising his drawing techniques. He had stopped drawing eight years earlier, at the time of his transition from theatre to cinema. Moreover, he had experimented with an unprecedented form of automatic writing, a tool associated with the expressive forms of surrealism, which allowed him to express the most intimate and uninhibited things that had been prompted by his contact with Mexico's history and culture.

This experience was a confirmation, for Eisenstein, of his idea – tuned with psychoanalysis and stimulated by his contacts with Vygotsky and Luria – that the effectiveness of art was connected to a regression towards pre-logical thinking. As Bordwell wrote: "His discussion of prelogical thought reflects his continuous affiliation with Vygotsky and Luria, who studied children, preliterate culture, and brain-damaged patients in search of cognitive processes at the variance of deductive reasoning" (Bordwell, 1993, p. 176).

This stream of thought was useful and congruent in artistic work, and we find traces of these ideas in the theoretical production of the second half of the 1930s and early 1940s. The issue of regression appears in the 1935 essay *The Film Form: New Problems*, written between 1935 and 1937, and in the texts collected for *Metod* and *Nonindifferent Nature*, written in the mid-1940s.

The connection between intrauterine regression, ecstasy and death is a subject which emerges in Eisenstein's Mexican drawings, which are full of symbols of anguish. Moreover, if we compare his film *Ivan the Terrible* (1944–1946) with Dostoevsky's novel *The Idiot* (1868–1869), Eisenstein refers to ecstasy, dealing with the topic of regression as a replication of a blissful state which corresponds to the "replication of the state of conception". Eisenstein outlines the same desire to return to the "matrix", to the original state, which is identified with the prenatal uterine state;

> Here the embryo develops in a completely autarkic dimension, standing still and closed in itself, free of all sensations from external influences, including the universal laws of attraction and the feeling of heaviness: this is the state of floating in the fluid element.
>
> *(Eisenstein, 2002, II, p. 302)*

These concepts, besides evoking Rank and Ferenczi's ideas, create a connection with the Freudian theory of narcissism. According to Freud's idea, during the intrauterine life and in the infant, the libido is directed towards the inner part of the individual, excluding the external world.

In the work *On Narcissism* (1914), Freud outlines the characteristics of this aspect of the psyche. Afterwards, elaborating on the second topography,[3] Freud designates the term primary narcissism a first stage of life before the constitution of the Ego, whose archetype is intrauterine life.

In a contemporary psychoanalytical perspective, this means an investment of the subject's libido, in other words, a failure to invest in the object. This implies that there is no separation between the subject and the external world.

Eisenstein is interested in this privileged condition, and he makes it overlap not only with the first phase of the individual's life but also, anthropologically, and biologically, with the most primitive moment of an ideal "evolution of the species".

On a philosophical and aesthetic level, the director wants to push viewers of works of art, films included, towards the dialectical unity of opposites, towards an art that is emotional and intellectual at the same time, towards a thought that is both logical and pre-logical.

This art advocates the synthesis of elements that the traditional mentality – embedded in logic and rationality – keeps separated. From an anthropological point of view, Eisenstein's personal contribution to anthropology is represented by the idea that the essence of the individual is made of these two opposing tendencies, with the conscious will clashing with an irrational and regressive non-will. On a methodological level, this contribution is based on psychological and psychoanalytical concepts. In fact, this was the topic of the lecture Eisenstein gave at the Berlin Psychoanalytic Institute in October 1929.

In these proposals, we see the echo of Freud's ideas who, in *Beyond the Pleasure Principle* (1920) – translated into Russian in 1925 – had associated the instinct of self-preservation and, more generally, the creative and conservative forces of the person to *Eros* and the regressive drives towards destruction and disaggregation to *Thanatos*.

In this work, Freud developed the notion of "repetition compulsion", according to which the subjects actively and repeatedly place themselves in conflictual and dreadful situations. In Freud's interpretation, the repetition compulsion is considered an independent factor which cannot be explained using only the principle of pleasure and the principle of reality. It is associated with a general characteristic of drives, to their conservative nature.

Drives have a conservative nature as they tend to restore an earlier state. This backward pattern leads the individual to death, following a process whereby inanimate matter, which becomes living, progressively tends to re-establish the inanimate state. On a conceptual level, it is a thermodynamic model; something like a progressive increase in entropy takes place, an echo of Sigmund Freud's nineteenth-century scientific mentality. Delving more deeply into the topic, differences will emerge.

While entropy represents the progressive decrease of a previous energetic drive, in the concept of Thanatos, there is a sort of independence, a drive which is a "push". In fact, Freud speaks of a "death drive", Thanatos, opposed by a "life drive", Eros, which is also biologically based. According to the father of psychoanalysis, sexuality is positioned at the basis of the Eros drive. It is worth mentioning here that the introduction to the Russian translation of Freud's volume *Beyond the Pleasure Principle* (1920) in 1925 was written by Vygotsky and Luria.

Eisenstein seems in tune with Freud's ideas and welcomes the co-presence of two opposing forces. This movement, by analogy, evokes the dialectical philosophical process. For this reason, he later claims that the creative work of art needs to be based on a dual movement: a visceral and regressive drive and, simultaneously, a progressive drive which leads towards higher layers of consciousness, and this can contrast the regression which is disruptive. Again, we find that there are no separate stages of development, individual and social, organised along a straight path towards higher levels.

As previously mentioned, the theory that regressive forces, individual and social, live by coexisting with developmental drives was, for Eisenstein, politically problematic. Somaini wrote:

> The importance Eisenstein attributed to all these "paths of regression" toward organic, psychological or social conditions characterized by a lack of differentiation, was in sharp contrast with a state ideology which was centered around the celebration of the conquests of a forward-moving socialism fighting against all forms of backward-oriented resistance. Eisenstein was well aware of this contrast.
>
> *(Somaini, 2016, p. 44)*

The Stalinist ideology of the state followed an interpretation of dialectics that tended to slip into mechanism. The "dialectical leaps" of human history were supposed to produce a new society where the past models of social functioning had to be conclusively erased and overcome. History was even attributed to an automatic "internal force" and a teleology tending relentlessly towards the realisation of socialism and, consequently, towards the configuration of human beings with positive characteristics, different from past humanity. In this way, the human "subjective factor" was mechanically subjugated to the dynamics of historical functioning, and this allowed Stalinist ideology to blame the individual and social "remains of the past" for all the failures, personal and collective, in the transformative push towards the new. Soviet society aimed to form a "New Man" in a "New World".

Stalin, like Lenin before him, had fully understood the social and political importance of cinema and had introduced cinematography in his first quinquennial plan. He had also fostered the construction of hundreds of cinemas across the Country and demanded the production of Russian cinema films and cameras which could be competitive with foreign technologies. Eisenstein was subject to direct criticism by the dictator. Between 1926 and 1929, Eisenstein had worked on *The General Line*, and in the Spring of 1929, the autocrat had examined the film. In that year, before he left to go abroad, Eisenstein was summoned to the Kremlin, along with Aleksandrov and Tissé. Stalin discussed cinema and Marxism and changed the film title from *The General Line* to *Old and New*. Still not satisfied, he suggested a different ending and planned an educative journey in the Russian fields for the three of them.

In the ideal Stalinist communist society, harmony was supposed to reign, and consequently, if something did not work, the responsibility was given to the resistance of what was "old". The director had different ideas; he cultivated the idea, which was labelled as anti-regime at the time, that the past, even if outdated, should not be rejected but re-elaborated and rethought in another and more complex stage of historical and social development.

It seems an adaptation, from top to bottom, of Heraclites' sense. In the work *General Theory of Montage*, Eisenstein writes:

> Only in the right age of his individual existence, of the existence of his species (social evolution) and of the existence of his society (the dialectical philosophy of mature humanity) does this separateness recomposes itself into a unity of renewed quality. The unilaterality of the *infant's* global thought becomes the conscious thought of the *adult*, which also incorporates the principle of differentiation. In so doing, the consciousness of man *at the dawn of culture*, becomes *the consciousness* of *man* in an *evolved age of culture. In the same way, philosophy becomes materialistic and dialectical out of primitive chaos*. Here, the following consideration is interesting: global perception is certainly the lower stage of perception (see Engels) while the differentiated perception is a step forward. The observation based on the *capacity for generalisation* is without any doubt the highest moment. (Thus, in science we talk of *universal concepts*, in art of *generalised images* but in both cases, we are at the highest level of man's spiritual activity, provided that both are consciously or intuitively directed towards the progressive growth or the transcendence of social reality, within the limits and directions traced by the social era they belong to). There seems to be a contradiction here: the highest level – the generalised image – due to its *plastic configuration* seems to coincide with the most primitive type of global perception. In fact, contradiction is only apparent; in this case we are facing that *precise* "almost-return to the past" defined by Lenin when he referred to the problem of the dialectic of phenomena. The fact is that the generalisation is *effectively global*, but it is such because it is a representation of the phenomenon (and the idea on the phenomenon) that is both global (immediate) and differentiated (mediated). If we deleted the individual figurative *element* from the generalisation, it would remain hanging as a bare, non-objectual abstraction.
>
> *(Eisenstein, 1985; Ital. transl., pp. 118, 119)*

In Engels' perspective, Eisenstein's aim remains connected to the philosophical dialectic, which sees the present and future as holding the signs of all that has already been.

The dialectical development characterises both human beings and the world around them, natural and artificial. Through its images impressed on film, cinema must strive to capture this development and foster it.

When Eisenstein gave a lecture at the official venue of the *Soviet Film Workers' Conference* in 1935, his ideas had an impact that went far beyond the debate on aesthetics and art. The goal of the conference was to validate the new doctrine of "socialist realism", and the director's ideas seemed to be a critique of the regime's theoretical framework, which aimed to overcome and erase the "bourgeois past". Another critical issue was the indirect references to the psychoanalytical theory. As previously mentioned, psychoanalysis had long been overtly opposed in the Soviet Union.

The idea that nothing in the life of human consciousness could be definitively overcome and forgotten was particularly controversial. In *Civilization and Its Discontents* (1929), Freud stated that "In mental life nothing which has once been formed can perish – that everything is somehow preserved and that in suitable circumstances (when, for instance, regression goes back far enough) it can once more be brought to light" (Freud, 1929; Engl. transl., p. 79).

According to Eisenstein, the inclination towards regression is a matter of fact which emerges in several parts of his work. That is how the activity of consciousness and the pattern which leads to the composition of art both work (see Angelini, 2020, pp. 218, 219).

In *Nonindifferent Nature* (1981), written between 1945 and 1947, employing a psychoanalytical term, Eisenstein defines as "introspective" the movement that allows individuals to "sink" into themselves. These are subjective feelings, but artworks, particularly cinema can enact this backward journey through the different stages of the development of consciousness.

In the first half of the 1940s, Eisenstein wrote:

> This means that the "method" of my "intellectual cinema" is based on the fact that from the most developed form of expression of consciousness the individual moves (backwards) to the most primitive form of consciousness… and here I am overcome by a worrying thought, a supposition. What if this transfer of the logical formula from the forms of the current level of our consciousness (in reverse!) to the form of the most primitive consciousness and thought is the secret of art in *general* (and not only of my "intellectual cinema")?
>
> *(See Eisenstein, in Bertetto P. ed., 1975, Ital. transl. pp. 223, 224)*

This tendency, perceived as universal, is present in any area of the director's interests. It corresponds to dialectical philosophy; every movement is always a double movement.

Film editing works in this way too; on the one hand, it unbundles what is given cinematically, reducing it to more elementary forms; on the other hand, it recomposes it at a higher, emotional and affective level of meaning.

In a passage from *Montaž* (*General Theory of Montage*, 1985, p. 169), he takes up, metaphorically, some themes which are discussed in Freud's *Totem and Taboo* (1913). The body of the tribe's chief, after being dismembered, was ideally reassembled in the collective ritual of the community. Similarly, montage leads first to the disassembling of the existing and then to a reassembling in a new and compact entity.

Through montage, cinema has the possibility to reconfigure reality in a linguistic and expressive sense. Here, Eisenstein takes from Vygotsky's ideas. The director sketches the construction of the language of images, using ideas from the concepts employed by the psychologist to describe human language functioning. The idea of "inner monologue" is fundamental.

Cinema works according to rules that do not belong to the rationality and logic that characterise external language in its oral and written forms. With concern to psychoanalytical ideas, the Freudian notion of *condensation* already emerged in some contributions written in 1929, such as *Dramaturgy of Film Form*. This idea is associated with the image, which condenses multiple contents. Eisenstein, in other words, believes that image is the most powerful tool to "grasp" phenomena and objects.

Image, in the work of artistic creation, allows the heterogeneity of different elements to a "condensed" vision (Eisenstein, 1986a; Ital. transl., p. 40). In Freudian thought, the concept of condensation represents one of the essential ways in which the unconscious processes function. A single representation sets, alone, different associative chains, and it represents their intersection point. On an economic level, it is invested by the sum of energies belonging to the different chains. Condensation is active in the symptoms and, in general, in the different formations of the unconscious, but most of all, it is active in dreams. In dreams, the manifest content is laconic and condensed compared to the latent content, and it represents a synthetic translation of it. Nevertheless, condensation is not a summary; it is determined by many latent meanings, and conversely, each meaning can be found in several elements.

In the essay *Vertical Montage* (1940a), Eisenstein introduces the possibility of a polyphonous montage where different components act "to create a *complex sentiment of the whole piece* … For music coordination, this *general sentiment* is extremely important because it is linked to the *sense of the totality of the image*, both musical and figurative" (Eisenstein, 1986; Ital. transl., p. 134).

Through different synchronised representations, above all the visual and the acoustic, the authentic sense of the *global image* emerges, and it is capable of conveying, in full strength, the *global content* of the work. In this ideal image, different pieces of the representation are condensed and combined vertically simultaneously. Vertical montage reaches its full ripeness on a conceptual level, in terms of concepts, in the more mature stage of Eisenstein's work (Angelini, 2020, p. 223).

After the Mexican experience, Eisenstein was overwhelmed by heterogenous stimuli transpiring different eras; he felt the need for a new aesthetic conception, less tied to the limits of causality and determination, a vision less restrained by the necessary and linear order of things. According to Cervini, this sentiment had

> a strong impact not only on his anthropological and psychological studies, but also on his aesthetic vision, for example on his last articulation of *vertical montage*. It is no coincidence that it never corresponds to a simple combination of images, connected on the ground of a presumed and realistic consequentiality of events. Of course, this had an impact on his interpretation of storytelling in its generality, not only in the field of cinema. What is challenged is the very idea of a tale narrated through images undermining a narrative model based on an analytical, logical, rationalistic vision of processes and temporal development. From a strictly literary point of view, this explains Eisenstein's passion for Joyce who had brought literature, according to Eisenstein, to a climax. With concern to the historical field, this leads to a detachment from a simple historicism, typical of some "vulgar exegetes of Marxism" and the decisive affirmation of what – according to Eisenstein – possesses the power and value of evidence: the idea, let us re-iterate, that history cannot progress in its development in a univocal way.
>
> *(Cervini, 2010, Ital. transl. p. 50)*

Regarding the concept of vertical montage, it is important to note that film montage in Eisenstein's time was carried out with the *moviola*, which is still used today for film montage. However, contemporary cinema is mostly shot with digital tools, and, in this case, film montage is done with computers.

Moviola allows one to see various parts of a film that one can then put together to compose the final product. Today filmmakers have different techniques at their disposal, but in Eisenstein's time, the rolled film was placed horizontally on the moviola and could slide forwards or backwards, but only horizontally. The idea of vertical montage, then, introduced an unexpected and innovative term, endowed with a symbolic value, aimed at describing an unprecedented action, primarily mental, which had to be then carried out with film and sound.

The vertical montage of the different shots brought the formation of ideas which were not conceivable in shots taken individually. It is not a matter of mere "additions" but overlays selected to create a *simultaneity* of different perceptual planes. The key idea is that, by virtue of this simultaneity, the emotion resulting from one piece overlaps the perceptive trace left by the previous one. In Eisenstein's ideas, we see the influence of the Freudian concept of condensation and the Vygotskyan notion of inner language agglutination (see Vygotsky, 1934, Chapter 7) that shall be further discussed.

The idea of verticality in montage can be understood, in a metaphorical sense, as a mental verticality, a montage that reaches, vertically, the archaic depths of the instinctual unconscious and simultaneously the higher zones of conscious thought. The aim is a synthesis of *sensual thought*.

If we look at the influence of Freud's psychoanalytical ideas on Eisenstein's theorisations and work, we should also mention the idea of displacement. In psychoanalysis, the term *displacement* essentially indicates a defence mechanism, the transfer of the interest and intensity of a representation, the transfer from one intense representation to a less intense one, connected to the first by an associative chain. This phenomenon is found, in particular, in the analysis of dreams but also in the formation of symptoms and, in general, in any construction of the unconscious.

From a psychoanalytical perspective, on a descriptive economic level, we assume that the energy of an investment separates from associations and flows along associative paths. The reason for this process is related to the *representability* of determined elements inside the psyche. In some cases, certain emotions related to desires or ideas are not *representable*. In dreams, it is the oneiric censorship that prevents representation. Therefore, only *displacement* can make those emotions and ideas representable through tangible oneiric images.

Eisenstein, in some early works, such as *Fuori campo* (*Offscreen*) and *Drammaturgia della forma cinematografica* (*The Dramaturgy of Film Form*, see Eisenstein, 1986), had talked about the topic in a strictly analogical manner. Even back then, his ideas focused on the possibility of representing – cinematically – abstract concepts, claiming that an abstract concept could be described by *transferring it* to a concrete image.

On a formal level, in a psychoanalytical sense, this also echoes the idea of *regression*. In fact, compared to structuration and differentiation, displacement outlines a passage to simpler ways of expression, as opposed to complexity. In dreams, regression transforms the motivations of emotions and the structures of thoughts into oneiric images. Dreams can be considered a regression that sets off primitive drives in the dreamer, opposing the progressive movement towards consciousness. According to Freud, additionally, dreams open a window into the phylogenetic infancy of human beings: "… we may expect that the analysis of dreams will lead us to a knowledge of man's archaic heritage, of what is psychically innate in him" (Freud, 1900, p. 549).

In this perspective, the connection to the sensitive thought of images does not characterise only one's dreams and childhood. Following this perspective, phylogenetically, at its primordial stage, humanity used this pattern of thinking. At a later stage, Eisenstein writes – showing the influence of Vygotsky – "Thought by images, which is a primitive form of thought, evolves into conceptual thinking" (Eisenstein, 1986; Ital. transl., p. 5). In thinking through images, Eisenstein looks for that primitive *sensory dimension*, mediated by ethnological studies and particularly by Lévy-Bruhl. This sensory dimension was imperative to him for defining art. In the Vygotskyan idea of inner monologue, Eisenstein aims to find evidence of the persistence of archaic forms of thought, even in the most developed structures of consciousness.

During the twentieth century and in more recent times, even in the specific field of psychoanalysis, the relationship between images and emotions from the perspective of the unconscious (see Kris, 1936; Metz, 1977; Deleuze, 1983; Angelini, 1992) was widely investigated. Ferruta (2005) has argued that

> The iconic configuration…is used to represent in images an emotion that is difficult to conceive, a proto emotion in search of representability which finds in the visual a way to make its way into the world of the subject's mind…reflection on thinking in images takes us to the heart of analytical functioning.
>
> *(Ferruta, 2005, p. 25)*

Hautmann (1993) had studied the characteristics of visual participation in the analytic situation and stated that visual participation in analysis is artificially reduced because of the setting. Ferruta (2005) delves into this idea, saying that

> the iconic imagination, in the resetting of perception, aided by the analytic setting, by the darkness in which dreams take shape and by the darkness of the cinema, outlines a specific level of mental functioning, which requires not to be obscured by other levels of symbolisation, capable of forming associations and centred on language. To reach thinkability certain emotions resort to the iconic as a path towards symbolisation, which activates new form of the container-contained relation to control an unthinkable emotion, translating it into a figure. This way of functioning belongs to the primitive mind, not in a chronological sense, but in terms of emotions that the subject is not able to contain and that, communicating with another mind – the analyst's mind – take on the dimension of figurability.
>
> *(Ferruta, 2005, p. 26)*

The topic of figurability of thought and emotions was an aspect discussed by the director on several occasions. In *Nonindifferent Nature*, showing a deep psychological insight, he wrote:

> In other words, if it is true that there is a stage of thought in which the concept (*ponjatie*) has not assumed a shape and the only instrument of expression is the image, we must also assume that there is an even more primal state, based uniquely on sentiment (*oscuscenie*), which is entirely devoid of means of expression other than mere symptoms of that state.
>
> *(Eisenstein, 1981; Ital. transl., p. 185)*

This statement paves the way to a reflection in which it is emphasised that any psychological "state" attains "concrete thematic objectivity" only through association with real objects. Reflecting on the necessarily historical nature of associations of this type, Eisenstein eventually dismissed any supra-historical, purely naturalistic hypothesis in the representation of human sentiments.

From the psychoanalytical perspective, through regression, the most elementary states of consciousness, inherent to humanity in its creation and typical of infantile behaviour, can reveal themselves at the highest levels of psychological development. This happens in different forms, in dreams and neurosis, according to Freud, and in art, according to Eisenstein. The "fundamental problem" that the director aims to examine when he begins writing *Metod* is related to these issues. In short, he wonders what the origin of creativity is and what are the qualities that enable the individual to have an expressive capacity, not only rational but also emotional, that takes the name of art.

It is also important to recall that Eisenstein's conceptual relation with psychoanalysis was neither fully linear nor devoid of conflictual nuances. On the contrary, in the latter part of his life, he criticised Freudian theory. He did not like the idea of a "violent" conflict between different layers of the psyche, such as the conscious and the unconscious, in conflicting forms.

He believed it was necessary to think of the complex life of consciousness in terms of unity and totality. When this connection between different higher and lower layers of consciousness does not work, it depends on an abnormal order, on something pathological; "It is interesting that this type of approach, developed as a reflection of an abnormal order of social facts, is convincing only if it deals with something pathological, organically abnormal, like a clinical case" (Eisenstein, 2002, vol. 1, p. 180).

Psychoanalysis has value in the pathological dimension, but its scarce "dynamism" makes it difficult to enter "the field of images".

This dynamic unity, an essential idea for Eisenstein, represents – in the philosophical dialectical perspective – a "synthesis". It was supposed to find its highest expression in art, and, on a historical and political level, it was supposed to translate into the construction of a socialist society. According to Eisenstein, it is in this dynamic aspect that psychoanalysis lacks adequacy. This limit is also reflected in the social dimension: "This deficiency depends mostly on the fact that Freud's perspective assumed an abnormal social development and did manifest the will to overcome it and was destined to end up interpreting certain phenomena in a wrong way" (Eisenstein, 2002, p. 181).

In general, while it is clear that psychoanalysis was one of the intellectual realities that mostly influenced Eisenstein, he was not adept. Like other leading artists of the early twentieth century, he welcomed and used psychoanalytical thought but, within certain limits, remained critical towards certain features. At the same time, he was also extremely interested in the general ideas of Russian psychology of that period. As illustrated, his first interests in biomechanics came from Meyerhold, his first mentor, and by the scientific work of Ivan Pavlov and Vladimir Bekhterev. On a historical level, however, Eisenstein's most important ideas, both from a psychoanalytical and a psychological perspective, came from the innovative ideas of Vygotsky.

Notes

1 For a complete chronology of the Russian translation of the main works of psychoanalysis during the first three decades of the twentieth century, see Angelini (1988), p. 41.
2 Letters from Sergei Eisenstein to Wilhelm Reich, in Ionin, 1977, (1), pp. 181–183.
3 The theory of the "psychical apparatus", or "topographical point of view" assumes a differentiation of this apparatus into a certain number of systems endowed with different characters and functions and arranged in a certain order; this allows to consider them metaphorically as psychical places and a spatial representation can be given of them. Two are the main Freudian 'topographies': in the first the main distinction is between unconscious, preconscious and conscious, and the second distinguishes three instances: Id, Ego, and Super-Ego.

5

EISENSTEIN AND VYGOTSKY'S PSYCHOLOGY

As already discussed, in his expressive maturity, Eisenstein was significantly influenced on a historical and conceptual level and from a psychological perspective by two great figures who were also his personal friends, Lev Vygotsky and Aleksandr Luria.

From a theoretical perspective, the most significant influence came from Vygotsky, one of the most representative scientific personalities of the time – the "Mozart" of twentieth-century psychology – whose studies gave rise to the cultural-historical theory and deeply influenced different and numerous areas of contemporary research: "Vygotsky made valuable contributions, from aesthetics to linguistics, from psychology to psychiatry" (Mecacci, 1986, p. 9). As discussed, for both Vygotsky and Eisenstein, the problem of methodology was a fundamental premise for undertaking any work.

In *Thinking and Speech* (1934), the first question Vygotsky raised concerned the most suitable method to address the "question of the relationship between thinking and speech". Vygotsky did not want to break psychological wholes into the elementary components that constituted them: from this perspective of analysis, thought and speech would not solve the problem due to the inability to preserve, in each element, "the characteristics of the whole";

> … a psychology that decomposes verbal thinking into its elements in an attempt to explain its characteristics properties will search in vain for the unity that is characteristic of the whole. These characteristics are inherent in the phenomenon only as a unified whole. When the whole is analysed into its elements, these characteristics evaporate. In his attempt to reconstruct these characteristics, the investigator is left with no alternative but to search for external, mechanical

DOI: 10.4324/9781003398554-6

> forms of interaction between the elements ... The contradictory nature of this form of analysis is clearly manifested in psychological research. Rather than providing an explanation of the concrete characteristics of the whole that we are interested in, it subordinates this whole to the dictates of more general phenomena. That is, the integral whole is subordinated to the dictates of laws which would allow us *to* explain that which is common to all speech phenomena or all manifestations of thinking, to speech and thinking as abstract generalities.
>
> *(Vygotsky, 1934; Engl. transl., p. 43)*

A similar critique had been already outlined in chapter eight of *The Historical Meaning of the Crisis in Psychology* (1927).

Vygotsky wondered: "What then is a unity that possesses the characteristics inherent to the integral phenomenon of verbal thinking that cannot be further decomposed? In our view, such unity can be found in the inner aspect of the word, in its meaning" (Vygotsky, 1934; Engl. transl., p. 44). Inside it, we can find a sense of the relation between thinking and speech because the meaning of a word is a *generalisation*, a way of reflecting reality that is different from how it is reflected in sensations and perceptions.

At this point, for the psychologist, there is a dialectical leap which is peculiar to human beings: the ability to generalise reality. Indeed:

> what distinguishes the basic unit – qualitatively and substantially – is the "generalised reflection of *reality*", generalisation in word meaning is an act of thinking in the true sense of the word. At the same time, however, meaning is an inseparable part of the word; it belongs not only to the domain of thought but to the domain of speech. A word without meaning is not a word, but an empty sound. A word without meaning no longer belongs to the domain of speech.
>
> *(Vygotsky, 1934; Engl. transl., p. 44)*

The phenomenon of generalisation favours the birth of speech and feeds the human tendency towards sociality. The acquisition of speech leads to that *dialectical leap* that allows the passage from the elementary, instinctual psychological functions to the higher functions of generalised thought. Outlining this passage, Vygotsky provides a dynamic representation of consciousness that contains an idea of development applied to the meaning of the word as a union of thinking and speech. Consciousness is always considered in its historical nature.

When Eisenstein began to speculate around a theory of montage, he had to think about a linguistic theory of cinema.

Intellectual cinema, seen as an expression of conscious, organised thought, is not consistent with the ideas of Vygotsky and with the psychoanalytical concept of the unconscious. The representation of emotions immediately leads to the question of the "inner monologue".

Vygotsky's studies referred to "inner speech" as a means of communication which is freer than the rigid constraints of ideally pure rational thought. This represented a solution for artistic problematic issues that had heavy philosophical implications.

Firstly, the need to overcome metaphysical, philosophical dualism that makes primary emotional functions irreconcilable with higher psychological functions, producing a fracture. On the other hand, Vygotsky claims the unitary and dynamic nature of consciousness. This translates, in psychological terms, into the necessity to achieve a concrete and not theoretical synthesis in which art and psychology can, at the same time, make mutual contributions.

The desire for such a synthesis was widely shared by leading figures like Eisenstein and Vygotsky, who supported the perspective of materialist dialectics. Psychology, which deals with consciousness, where emotions and thoughts coexist, could have used more aspects of this synthesis. Eisenstein's idea of a "unitary double movement" manifested and realised this synthesis in art, materialising with the "simultaneous penetration", both upwards and downwards, of the psyche.

The perspectives of both the psychologist and the director were common because they methodologically based their research on the paradigm of dialectical materialism. The philosophical belief that developments in nature and social history advance by *qualitative*, not only *quantitative*, brought Vygotsky to take distance from the Pavlovian "stimulus-response" scheme, which outlined a purely mechanical model of human functioning.

The dimension of quality, which is proper to dialectics, is alien to mechanism. Eisenstein aims for an organic conception of the work of art, which involves dialectics. With the term *organicity*, we refer to the adaptation to the laws that regulate the existence of nature and history, which are themselves dialectical. But it is necessary to define the relationship between subjectivity and objectivity, between inside and outside, which must always be understood as a dynamic product. In both psychology and art, the dynamism of the dialectical process determines the evolutionary process that leads to the generation of both consciousness and art. For Vygotsky, already in *The Psychology of Art* (1925a), the research for laws that could explain the functioning of consciousness is aligned with the research for laws that could explain the functioning of artistic processes.

In the same period, Aleksandr R. Luria, one of the founders of contemporary neuropsychology and a supporter of Vygotsky's ideas, was a close friend of Eisenstein's and promoted various educational and research projects with him. The lives of Luria and Eisenstein intertwined for great part of the director's life in the name of a great friendship.

Luria quoted Eisenstein in his work on the notorious mnemonist S.V. Šereševskij (Luria, 1968), recalling the interest of the director in the phenomenon of synaesthesia in the clinical events of this man with an exceptional memory. For the same reason, Eisenstein mentioned Šereševskij in his work. Nevertheless, Eisenstein's name does not appear in Luria's autobiography, which is full of prominent figures related to Russian culture and science.

Mecacci (2011) believes that this was due to the fact that for a long time, the psychologist carefully avoided references to personal events, not out of modesty and privacy, but out of a "political" choice with regard to sensitive issues. In this specific case, because of the still looming anti-Semitism, which was rekindled in 1948 and culminated in the repression of Jewish doctors between 1952 and 1953 accused of having assaulted the Soviet state.

Additionally, there was the attack on pro-bourgeois and Western cultural orientations, and those who showed even the slightest interest in psychoanalysis were consequently attacked, "guilty" of being born and being rooted in Western culture, in the Jewish world, and within the bourgeois class.

Historically, the relationship between Eisenstein and Luria became known to scholars of Russian psychology and linguistics after the second edition of Vygotsky's *The Psychology of Art* in 1968. For this second edition, the text was adjusted considering Vygotsky's typescript, on which the first edition of 1966 was based, and another typescript copy, containing some pen and ink corrections by Vygotsky himself.

This typescript copy was in Eisenstein's personal archive and was discovered by Naum I. Kleiman. The new edition of Vygotsky's *The Psychology of Art* contained an extraordinary commentary by linguist Viacheslav V. Ivanov. The latter returned on several occasions to the theoretical relations between the Vygotskyan school and the Russian director and on his project to give life to a systematic collaboration with Vygotsky and Luria to study film in its psychological dimension.

In his 1976 work on Russian semiotics, Ivanov shed light on the influence of psychology on Eisenstein's work. This work became a reference point for the different studies on the interaction between Vygotskyan psychology and Eisenstein's aesthetics. Luria continued to support and give advice to Eisenstein in the field of psychology for all his life. In November 1947, the director, "upon request of A.R. Luria", began to collect notes on the psychology of art, which he had been gathering since 1940. He also prepared a list of lectures to give on this subject at the Moscow Institute of Psychology for his friend's students, and probably Luria gave Eisenstein Vygotsky's typescript *The Psychology of Art*.

Unfortunately, Eisenstein did not accomplish the task because he died on the night between the tenth and eleventh of February 1948. Here is the painful evocation of the director's passing by Luria's daughter, Elena, with a mention of the "terrible years" of Stalinism:

> Sergei Mikhailovich's death was a disaster for our family. I remember that my father asked me to go into his study and I sat down next to him on the sofa and, in a flat voice, unusual in him, he slowly said: "Sergei Mikhailovich died last night" ...Through the window I could see a grey winter day, and my father's

study was half-darkened. Before my eyes I saw beams of coloured sparks and a sort of electricity run through my body, as had happened to me when I stuck scissors in a socket as a child. My father looked calm and concentrated. As I understood later, he never showed his pain to others; in those sad minutes he did not say anything strong, the pain was inside him...Sergei Mikhailovich was a friend to my father, they were bound together by many things and by the delight of an intellectual relationship. They faced together difficult years when people were afraid to speak frankly even with their wives. In those terrible years (after the end of the war) Eisenstein showed my father the manuscripts of the great film director Meyerhold, who had been arrested in 1939. Following the arrest, Meyerhold's archive was hidden in Eisenstein's *dacha* on the second floor, in the wooden cupboard, and I saw them, my father and Sergei Mikhailovich, putting those files in order. After Sergei Mihajlovic's death, my father arranged for Eisenstein's brain to be preserved after the autopsy. They put it in a large glass container, in formalin. My father took this glass container home and put it on a cold table, which we used as a refrigerator in winter. At the time, I did not know it; I only noticed that *Olya* (short for Olga, her mother) was bothered and unhappy about something. One evening I saw the large glass container on the table and noticed there was something like the kernel of a gigantic walnut. It struck my interest, and I lifted the lid and smelled a strong smell that lingered in my nose for a while and then took my breath away. I closed the container and ran to my mother: "Olya, what is that there?" She did not answer, she only said irritated talking to herself: "I told him that he can't keep this thing in the house!" Later that evening I learned from my father that it was Sergey Mihajlovic's brain. He told me that the brain of a genius should be preserved for science. But I burst into tears and asked it to be taken out of the house...Eisenstein's brain is kept at the Brain Institute in Moscow, but in our archive, there are *photographs* and other things on Sergey Mikhailovich: his manuscripts, drawings, recordings of interviews and the texts of my father's lectures on him.

(Luria E., 1994, pp. 127, 128)

Eisenstein was buried in the Novodevichy Cemetery in Moscow, in a grave close to that of Vygotsky.

Since the 1920s, Luria considered Eisenstein an exemplary figure within the context of the Muscovite culture, a culture which was imbued with psychoanalysis, with prominent figures who disappeared during the period of Stalinism and of whom there would be no news until the early 1990s, after the dissolution of the Soviet Union.

Chronologically, it is difficult to say the exact period in which Eisenstein met Vygotsky and Luria. According to Luria's daughter (1994, p. 120), her father began seeing the director between the end of 1925, after the premiere of *The Battleship Potemkin* on the 25th of December, and the beginning of 1926.

During a lecture given on the 19th of February 1962 at Moscow University (Mecacci, 2011, p. 103), Luria recalled he went to Eisenstein's house to discuss psychological issues rather than cinema; in particular, they discussed the relationship between expression and creativity. Luria's interest in film, theatre and art in general was also encouraged at that time by his relationship with his first wife, Vera N. Blagovidova, who was a theatre actress.

Their marriage lasted from 1923 to 1929. At the end of the 1920s, Luria undertook a series of experiments with Eisenstein on the imagination of movement using hypnosis. What follows is the transcript of an experimental session conducted with the director:

> Test protocol 13/12/28.
>
> Experimental subject M.I.

A circular movement from left to right is suggested, which is meant to recall a circular walk in the Alupkinsky Park [a vast park in the city of Alupka, southern Crimea]. The circular movement should be repeated twice, with half-closed eyes, without perceiving the surroundings. The subject at the given signal stands up, goes to the next room, and starts to move in a circle.

Experimenter: "In the middle of the field, there is a column with something". The subject stares at the centre of the circle, slows down and immediately moves towards the centre of the spiral.

Experimenter:

> Look at the beautiful pear on the column. You are very thirsty, and you want to take the pear… You hesitate, fearing that a wasp might sting you… But the desire wins… You decide to take the pear… You keep an eye on it and go into the other room. The wasp has flown away…
>
> *(quoted in Mecacci, 2011, p. 103)*

The experiments were aimed at studying how the mind could imagine and reproduce a real situation with relative movements, a psychological phenomenon that interested the director. In these sessions, hypnosis was induced by Juri V. Kannabikh (1872–1939), an expert in the technique and a prominent figure in Russian psychiatry and psychoanalysis in the first three decades of the century. At the time of his participation in Luria and Eisenstein's experiments, Kannabikh was the president of the Russian Psychoanalytical Society, and he would be the last since the Society was closed in 1930.

At the beginning of 1910, Kannabickh had founded a clinic for mental illnesses in Kryukovo, near Moscow, where patients were treated with psychotherapy, psychoanalytical techniques, and the use of hypnosis. It was a very famous clinic in which well-known exponents of Russian culture and art were treated for psychological disorders, such as the poets Aleksandr A. Blok and Sergei M. Solovev, the actor Mikhail A. Chekhov, Anton's nephew, and the theatre director Evgenii B. Vakhtangov.

One of the psychotherapists who worked in the clinic was Aron B. Zalkind. Kannabickh had also been the therapist of Adolph A. Ioffe, one of the main protagonists of the Bolshevik Revolution, head of the Military Revolutionary Committee, close friend of Trotsky and the leader of the Trotskyist opposition. In 1927, Ioffe committed suicide when his group began to be attacked and persecuted. Ioffe had also been in analysis, in Wien, with Alfred Adler and continued his therapy with Kannabickh. Eisenstein experienced various hypnosis sessions with Kannabickh, between 1935 and 1937 to treat depressive feelings that inhabited him since his return to the USSR after his American journey.

Trotsky and Ioffe were the two most prominent politicians to promote psychoanalysis in Russia. They conceived it as a revolutionary movement that could contribute to the birth of the new man. The support of psychoanalysis by the Trotskyists was the main historical reason for the ostracism of psychoanalysis in Russia, which manifested in the second half of the 1920s.

We know for sure that during the preparation of the film *October* (*Ten Days That Shook the World*), before 1928, Eisenstein had gathered a friendly "team" with Vygotsky and Luria, also including the linguist Nicolaj J. Marr. They discussed the topics of film art from an aesthetic and psychological perspective. These friends helped Eisenstein a lot in the mid-1930s while he was facing a great crisis.

In Bordwell's words:

> By the early 1930s Nikolai Marr had become the most influential Soviet linguist. Eisenstein was susceptible to Marxism. Marr's "stadial" theory of language change, whereby vocal language develops on the basis of manual or gestural sign systems, would have struck a sympathetic chord in the theatre director who thought of expressive movement as more basic than language. Marr's theory further posited a link between the origin of speech and the development of work processes ... Eisenstein's 1935 talk, delivered only a year after Marr's death, announces that Marr's theories have a methodological value beyond the field of linguistics ... Eisenstein calls upon the model of sensual thought [according to the original Russian expression, *chuvstvennoe myshlenie*, "sensual thinking" – our note] throughout his later theorizing. Sometimes he seeks to show the power of nonlogical formal choices. More often he stresses that concrete representational qualities of art tap prelogical processes, so that the most advanced and effective works combined knowledge of the conceptual implications of a phenomenon with a strongly sensuous formal appeal.
>
> *(Bordwell, 1993, p. 172)*

The reason Vygotsky and cultural-historical theory were so important in Eisenstein's intellectual evolution is that, conceptually, the Vygotskyan perspective and

Eisenstein's theoretical and artistic research direction were akin. Based on dialectical materialism, the use of a method capable of examining, in general, the philosophy of history and, at the same time, the relationship of the individual with the world is legitimised. Psychologists study thinking and emotion in their psychological dimension, and filmmakers are interested in thinking and emotion in the artistic dimension. From a philosophical point of view, speech and art are philosophically *moving forms* of human expression.

Art is supposed to activate, dialectically and simultaneously, the primitive and rational strata. In elaborating on secret, hidden layers of the psyche, the director links up with *sensual thinking* in the anthropological perspective outlined by Lévy-Bruhl (1910, 1922, 1931).

By following this pattern, which exalts the affective and instinctual aspects of the psyche, film editing is an effective tool to grasp the spectator. This is a quite different position compared to the criteria of intellectual montage used by Eisenstein, only a few years before his journey to Mexico, to express concepts through images. Montage related to *sensual thinking* is an analogous version of Vygotskyan inner monologue. It represents the third milestone of a journey that begins with the montage of attractions and passes through an intellectual montage. We should not forget that the content of concepts is, for Eisenstein, both *ideological* and *affective*. According to Eisenstein, knowledge is not a mere intellectual fact. As he writes in *Montage*, knowledge is gained through "the living interplay of passions" (Eisenstein, 1986a; Ital. transl., p. 220). This need for cinema – an excellence among the arts – to contain dialectically opposing forces equals the effort made by inner speech. The latter is set in the subject's mind in a dialectical relation between the verbal expression that tends to make it manifest and the emotion and will that sustain it on the level of psychological motivation. Artwork must reply to the expressive tools of inner speech, and cinema is not only "the most advanced of the arts" but also "the method of cinema, when fully comprehended, will enable us to reveal an understanding of the method of art in general" (Eisenstein, 1949, p. 194).

In the attempt to detect and expose the emotional dimension of cinema, even in concrete terms, Eisenstein was always close to psychoanalytical ideas. Etkind wrote:

> *Strike*, *October*, and *Potemkin* are full of scenes of mass panic and violence, scenes that could have been used as illustrations in Freud's "Group Psychology and Analysis of the Ego" (with which Eisenstein must have been familiar), if not for the opposite emotional timbre in which they were shot. Unlike Freud, Eisenstein felt no aversion to mass hypnosis; on the contrary, he felt drawn to melt into the crowd, and he invited his mass audience to join him.
>
> *(Etkind, 1993, p. 319)*

The sphere of *sensual thinking*, that part of the psyche that Eisenstein perceived as closer to instincts and emotions, faced its moment of greatest expression during his journey to Mexico. In his Mexican drawings, this is intensely expressed through the eroticism and pain they reveal. The period of the journeys to the USA and Mexico was, for Eisenstein, extremely intense and psychologically exhausting. In fact, in the USA, he had a short personal experience of psychoanalysis, as had previously occurred in Russia with Aron Zalkind. In Hollywood, he sought the help of a psychoanalyst, and it was Charlie Chaplin who suggested he contact Dr Cecil Reynolds.

Eisenstein wanted to overcome the difficulties that emerged during the realisation of a long-planned project which he never completed, *The Glass House*. In that period, Eisenstein was accompanied by Ivor Montagu, an interesting figure in the history of cinema, who worked in the production and montage of the filming.

Montagu was shocked to see Eisenstein "who began to spend hours – and cash – sitting with Dr. Reynolds on our balcony being analysed to find out the obstruction that prevented *him*, himself, from thinking of a 'Glass House' story" (Montagu, 1968, p. 105). This was only Montagu's opinion, and we do not know what came out of these sessions.

It must be said that Montagu considered Eisenstein's *The Glass House* a sort of obsession, a kind of addiction. The film was based on the short story by Evgeny I. Zamyatin *We* (1919–1921), portraying a transparent world where houses are transparent, without walls to hide things, but the inhabitants do not see the walls are transparent and live as if they are not. It must be noted that the very same idea resurfaced in the film *Dogville* by Lars von Trier in 2003 in a different dramaturgical context. In this film, the streets and houses of the village, including interiors, are marked with white lines drawn on the ground, without walls or doors and with very little furnishing.

In producing a Hollywood version of Zamyatin's short story, Eisenstein wanted to make a satire of the socialist paradise, expressing the strong resistance of a man against mass society, which had deprived him both of his individuality and the feeling of love. It was a sign of Eisenstein's hard reaction against the distortions and mistakes of the Soviet world. The creator of *October* and *Battleship Potemkin* wanted to take advantage of his stay abroad to express a new, more critical attitude towards the regime in his country, but the result was a very intense inner ambivalence that ended up in an artistic block.

The reaction was probably due more to the perceived need to embrace a new and problematic vision of himself and the Soviet world than a form of homeland nostalgia. We can only imagine the overwhelming mixture of creative energy, fear of the regime, muddled ideas, and devotion to ideals that Dr Reynolds had to face while listening to this patient on the terrace of that Californian villa.

Eisenstein went back home in 1932. His contract to make the film *Qué viva Mexico!* was cancelled by the American commissioner due to pressure from the Soviet authorities. Back in Moscow, Eisenstein did not find the same positive atmosphere he had left almost three years earlier. It was as if he had to be punished for the freedom he had enjoyed and had to get back into the severe ranks of control to which all artistic production, not just cinema, was subjected, being controlled by centralised state structures. It was the period in which people started to talk about the so-called "socialist realism" introduced by Andrei Zhdanov during the *First Congress of Socialist Writers* in 1934. Eisenstein's film projects were stopped, and he accepted to go into teaching at the State Institute of Cinematography and work on his theoretical work. In 1935, as already mentioned, he took part in the All-Union Creative *Conference* of *Soviet Film Workers*, which aimed to extend the directives of socialist realism to cinema. In his essay *Film Form: New Problems* (1935), he suggested a compromise. On the one hand, he accepted socialist realism in general and underlined the continuity between the research of that time and research conducted in the late 1920s on intellectual cinema. Admittedly, even then, his aim was to bring "emotional fullness" to an ideologically oriented cinema. On the other hand, he shed light on the "new problems" that film form had to face.

In the essay, he talks about the pre-logical thought that, according to Lévy-Bruhl (1910, 1922, 1927), characterised knowledge in the context of "primitive mentality". In this perspective, we should collocate his ideas on the inner monologue. He suggests, as an example, James Joyce's use of language in *Ulysses*. It must be noted, however, that the concept of inner monologue is generated by his interest in the phenomenon of inner speech, introduced and studied by Vygotsky. The juxtaposition of the two terms, *inner monologue* and *inner speech*, is not casual, of course.

In the same year, 1935, Eisenstein resumed his creative work on the film *Bežin lug* (*Bezhin Meadow*). Filmmaking stopped in 1936, for the first time, due to an intervention by the Central Direction of Cinematography, requiring script changes. In 1937, due to a second intervention, Eisenstein had to stop working on the film. He was forced to write a severe self-critique, and the only existing copy of the film was confiscated and destroyed during the war.

This event brought Eisenstein into a state of emotional distress, making him think about the idea of "eliminating art", defining it as a "shameful activity". Cervini (2010), speculating on this crisis, points to the director's sorrow with how his earlier proposal of "intellectual cinema" had been sophisticated and extreme, advocating rationality and organised thought as the basis and subjects of films. Instead, the director's commitment towards the expressive possibilities of cinema was increasingly directed to the emotional component of thought, aspiring to break free from the strict and rational limits of intellectual cinema. Moreover, the linguistic rationality and the linearity of intellectual cinema were very distant from Vygotsky's idea of "inner speech" and from the "inner monologue" that Eisenstein was elaborating.

This was one of the most difficult periods in his life. Attacks from filmmakers that were politically aligned and from cultural bureaucrats became more and more violent and direct, and there was also the risk of deportation.

While Eisenstein was working on his most important theoretical texts during these years, which were later collected in *Montage*, written in 1938, he had many interior doubts. He was subject to criticism from outside, and, in this circumstance, he questioned the very possibility of continuing with filmmaking, both internally and externally. Eisenstein considered the idea of abandoning cinema. Recalling those years, he mentioned the great professional and personal help he received from the cultural and human exchange with Vygotsky and Luria;

> In very profound tones, the departed Vygotsky had tried to dissuade me from the intent, if not to destroy art, to abandon that shameful activity. I was very fond of that extraordinary man, as a scientist and as a person, with his very odd haircut. It always seemed as if his hair was growing back after typhus or one of those diseases for which one had to shave the head. Beneath that bizarre haircut, the most brilliant psychologist of our time looked at the world with his eyes of celestial clarity and transparency. Those eyes shone with sadness when he tried to make me abandon my evil intentions, which I expressed by addressing the most disdainful epithets of the sacred art. I also owe to a third person, a friend who is still enjoying good health, A.R. Luria, who introduced me to many of the mysteries of experimental psychology, usually not accessible to ordinary people. At a certain point, problems related to the emerging cinematographic language (especially with concern to the film *October*) had to be analysed in a systematic way by our "not bad at all team": Aleksandr Romanovich Luria, Vygotsky, Marr… Yes, exactly Nikolai Yakovlevich Marr and me… We began our work, but early death took two of us away. Now I am filming at Alma-Ata. Luria is treating with impressive results aphasics in a clinic near Chelyabinsk. Both attempts to dissuade me did not have an effect. I was saved by three circumstances.
>
> Lenin's words.
>
> A quotation by Engels.
>
> And above all, of course, my coming back from a Western society – condemned to philosophical dualism – to a country where monism triumphed in its highest emerging form, i.e., a state in which social class spirit had been erased. Emotionally detached from this monistic atmosphere, during the two years wandering the dualistic world that surrounded my country, in my theoretical awareness I had reached a very desolating conclusion, a torn idea, torn with the same noise made by the temple veil tearing itself from top to bottom in the tragic event on Golgotha. At the time even the tragic "interior torment of the soul" appeared to me like a Golgotha. I was saved by dialectics or, rather, by Lenin's words on the essence of dialectics.
>
> *(Eisenstein, 2020; Ital. transl., pp. 222–224)*

The reference to language problems caused by *October*, made to celebrate the tenth anniversary of the revolution, recalls an exceedingly difficult moment in the director's life. The film became a favourite target of Stalinist critics. The film featured technical experiments and used, like *Battleship Potemkin*, the criterion of synecdoche; it contained, for example, details of the objects of tsarist luxury, such as paintings, crockery, and furniture and symbols of the old world. Their destruction symbolised the victory of the proletariat: on one side, there were objects. On the other, there was a man. The film was not immediately understood by the public and was condemned by the critics. Moreover, it featured the figure of Lenin talking to the crowd, and this shot annoyed Mayakovski as he was contrary to any form of rhetoric.

In the mentioned passage by Eisenstein, the references to Lenin, Engels, and monist philosophy are worth our attention. However, there are a few sentences that testify how Eisenstein, even emotionally, felt the urge for methodological rigour as a premise for any enterprise, be it artistic or scientific. The image of a country where monist thought triumphed, surrounded "by the Western Countries, condemned by dualist philosophy" is almost blatant. In fact, it was not due to dialectical materialism that Eisenstein was hampered in his activity but because of the mechanistic drift of the Stalinist regime theorists.

In Russia, psychoanalysis faced a similar destiny for the same reason. Psychoanalysis, due to its early persecution, had no time to fully approach the heritage of Engel's dialectical materialism. The evolution of psychoanalytical thought in Western Countries eventually demonstrated that Eisenstein's fears related to the potential damage of the "dualist thought" were not groundless. Western psychoanalysis, in the last century, fragmented into small threads that, in their varied multiplicity, often resembled ideologies or, worse, mere opinions.

Eisenstein's friends Vygotsky and Marr died prematurely in 1934, but the director continued to meet Luria till his own death in February 1948.

Among others, Homskaya wrote on their friendship and collaboration;

> During the 1940s Luria kept in close touch with the famous film director S. M. Eisenstein, who made such masterpieces of world cinema such as *Potemkin* and *Ivan the Terrible*. Since becoming acquainted in the 1920s, Luria and Eisenstein shared a common interest in the psychology of art, and psychological aspects of artistic expressivity ... At the end of the 1920s, Luria organised an international association of scientific cinema and created a laboratory at the Institute of Cinematography to execute various kinds of cinematic shooting for scientific purposes ... In the 1930s, Luria and Eisenstein continued to exchange letters. Their correspondence continued during the Kharkov period and during the war. After the war, and until Eisenstein's sudden death in 1948, they often met, shared books, and talked.
>
> *(Homskaya, 2001, p. 39)*

The director was interested in the way psychoanalytical thought, amid false starts and interruptions, was developing a theory of art. Furthermore, in that period, Kris (1936) elaborated the idea of "regression in the service of the ego" within the domain of creativity. Kris was originally an art historian and advanced the idea that the ego, starting from the secondary process, could reach higher levels of functioning thanks to the capability to regress and draw on the greater richness of the primary process.

With concern to the psychoanalytical meaning of art, historically, psychoanalysis has often slipped into two pre-established positions, both questionable. In one case, a repertoire of fixed images and situations was created and used to provide universal theoretical interpretations. In the other case, the artist was clinically placed on an imaginary couch, and his creations were connected to his life. The first case shows a scholastic approach, and the second is a hagiographic one.

The collection of notes by Eisenstein, begun in 1940 and continued until 1947 under the title *Psychology of Art*, was destined for Luria's students, and it portrayed remarkably interesting considerations on methodology. Written by a mature Eisenstein, this work illustrates how, according to the director, a psychological interpretation of art is inherently connected to methodological criteria drawn from Marxism-Leninism. In his own words, "If we look at the history of art, it is in our time that three new elements emerge, which never existed before, and which provide useful prerequisites for shedding light on the question.

- Marxist-Leninist Methodology, which nurtures dialectical analysis of phenomena.
- Our social structure; a society without social classes, unprecedented in the history of humanity, since (with the end of primitive society) a pre-class social system ceased to exist.
- The echo of this arrangement in the superstructures provides unprecedented models, both in creative practice and in theoretical cognition. This has given life to a new pattern of thinking, which had never existed before, associated with art and with the formulation of questions related to art" (Eisenstein, 1940b, p. 2).

Like Vygotsky, Eisenstein elected Marxism and dialectic as a universal methodology that could be used in every field of knowledge. As previously stated, the director was influenced by his psychologist friend not only in his ideas on montage and inner monologue but, more generally, on the methodological and philosophical level. In this methodological perspective, cinema becomes "the most complete instrument of art". However, these ideas are also the result, speaking in Vygotskyan terms, of a social and cultural dimension that promotes this perspective;

> The cinematographic method is like a magnifying glass through which the method of all the arts becomes manifest. The method of all arts put together is the fundamental method of any form of art. Without the Marxist-Leninist method, without the actual social development and finally, without this sublime creation of human ingenuity and technology, still so little used, that is cinema, we would not be able to observe with such precision the most secret organism of form.
>
> *(Eisenstein, 1940b., p. 3)*

In *Psychology of Art* (1940b), the director, continuing to use general methodological ideas, moves to more concrete issues on a political level, like property and labour force, defending the Soviet social perspective. At the same time, he picks anthropological concepts that he had used to describe emotion in primitive art and the persistence of some archaic traits in contemporary superior artistic forms.

As written by Vyacheslav V. Ivanov,

> The affinity of Eisenstein with Vygotsky's ideas consisted in the fact that Eisenstein, differently from the ethnologists (anthropologists) and linguists (Lévy Bruhl and Marr) who were influential in his own thinking – who connected with absolute certainty pre-logical thought to ancient times or archaic societies – was interested in the expression of these ideas in relation to the life and art of contemporary man. Eisenstein found in our everyday behaviour the signs of the same structure of thought …And these conclusions are intertwined with the research that Vygotsky was carrying out at the time he began working with Eisenstein in the 1930s and which was published, for the first time, in 1960.
>
> *(Ivanov, 1977, pp. 328, 329)*

Vygotsky began his theoretical work starting with the structural organisation of the work of art, what we would call today "Reception Theory", that is to say, the effect art produces in the observer. Vygotsky's 1925 PhD thesis was entitled *Psychology of Art*, the same title used by Eisenstein for his work.

Vygotsky's *Psychology of Art* (1925a) retains several ideas that use the psychoanalytical perspective. Freud is quoted dozens of times, along with other authors such as Rank and Jung. The work was published in Russian in 1956 and translated into English only in 1971, but Eisenstein had a copy of the manuscript in his library and had read it carefully, as the thick notes on the margin testify. Eisenstein always strived to find a method to evoke specific answers in the receiver of a work of art and, particularly, in cinema spectators. This objective has been evident ever since his first idea of "Montage of Attractions", a work that he had begun when he was still in the theatre as a student of Meyerhold.

"Montage of Attractions" is a model aimed to produce a physiological effect. It is not important how stylised or distant from the real world the product is; what is important is its capability to stimulate and produce physical effects on the spectator. If the impact on the public is the aim, the formal organisation of the performance is the means. The form must tend to stimulate the spectator, and the basic element of this stimulation is "attraction".

The idea of attraction draws from the attractions of an imaginary circus or an amusement park. As Bordwell highlights,

> the sideshow, the roller coaster, the acrobatic turn… the attraction is thereby defined functionally, not substantively … Anything that jolts the spectator's sensory apparatus counts as an attraction, regardless of source or artistic status: Romeo's soliloquy, the color of an actress' tights, a drumroll. Traditional theatre buries its attractions within a plot structure … Attractions can be manifested in

setting, lighting, or any other aspect of the theatre (including firecrackers under the seats of the audience, as in *The Wiseman*).

(Bordwell, 1993, p. 117)

According to the theory of montage of attractions, cinema and theatre should be used as tools aimed to stimulate emotional reactions in the spectators, artistically and ideologically oriented. To pursue this objective, it is necessary to create a film montage that breaks away from mere naturalism to incorporate heterogeneous elements. Attractions are actions in theatre and images in cinema, randomly chosen and autonomous, but with a precise orientation, to achieve a specific final thematic effect. Cinema, Eisenstein believed, seemed particularly suitable, more than theatre, for the method of attractions, and he later became convinced that the global regeneration of dramaturgical space – his aspiration – could only be achieved through cinema.

His first film *Strike!* (1924–1925) represents an experiment on a montage of attractions with the aim, in a wider sense, to establish the aesthetical autonomy of cinema, rejecting any expressive dependence of this new tool on literary or theatrical models. In his following films, his idea of montage is consolidated and integrated. In *Battleship Potemkin* (1925), the "pathetic" sense of montage is intensified.

According to Van Der Veer "Eisenstein single-handedly originated a new style of filming with his *Battleship Potemkin*" (Van Der Veer, 2007, p. 24). In the film *October* (1927), the "intellectual perspective" prevails. In those years, Eisenstein had fluctuated, for a long time, between a "sensual" and a rational conception of montage. In his following work, he sought a greater balance between the two directions, even at a time when Stalinist authority strongly conditioned work, as we can see in his fourth film, *Old and New* (1929). The latter is considered by Etkin, from another perspective, evidence that "leaves no doubt" about the use of psychoanalysis in Eisenstein's work:

Eisenstein's intellectual engagement with psychoanalysis periodically waxed and waned according to the level of interest and the intensity of his resistance; but he continued to be involved with it throughout his life. Pavlov, Freud, and Meyerhold are the first three individuals mentioned in his huge autobiography; through the works of these writers, he undertook his youthful "joust with the windmills of mysticism". Eisenstein first read Freud in spring of 1918, while serving as a volunteer in the newly created Red Army … F. M. Ermler, a young actor who was close to Eisenstein in the 1920s and who would later become a famous director, remembered that Eisenstein knew Freud "with the usual systematic thoroughness that characterized his intellect"; according to him, scenes from the film *New and Old* leave no doubt that Eisenstein used psychoanalysis in his work…Eisenstein was friends with Stefan Zweig, who was in Russia not long before he wrote the book *Healing and the Psyche*, which contains a long, adoring anecdote about Freud. Zweig described Freud to the director as the

> "great Viennese", the "patriarch of the new Athenian School". Eisenstein wryly recalled how these stories "melded Plato and Aristotle into the overwhelming personality of the man with the Wagnerian first name". Zweig could not resist introducing Eisenstein to Freud, and in 1929 the latter agreed to a meeting in Vienna. The meeting never took place. Later, in 1946, Eisenstein described his analytic experience as "my raids into the fantastic jungles of psychoanalysis, jungles penetrated by the powerful breath of the *lebeda*". Lebeda, Russian for goosefoot, was Eisenstein's pun on Freud's concept of the libido.
>
> *(Etkind, 1997, pp. 315, 316)*

The theoretical work he left was partially published by Vjacheslav V. Ivanov (1976).

Eisenstein believed that the different criteria for the effectiveness of artwork functioned simultaneously, on several levels, within the work itself. This produced, in the mind of the viewer, a broader structural organisation, reaching both emotional and intellectual effects.

In the artistic work, the union of emotions and intellect was consistent with Vygotsky's ideas in terms of psychological concepts. For Vygotsky, the separation between the dimension of feelings and that of intellect represented a fundamental loophole in the traditional psychology of the time (Vygotsky, 1927).

The Vygotskyan vision indicates the existence of a dynamic system of consciousness, where affectivity and intellect are to be seen in their mutual dependence. Vygotsky's appreciation for psychoanalysis is related to the fact that this discipline tends to adhere to this criterion. From this perspective, even and especially the emotions that come from art are to be conceived as "intelligent emotions".

On a biographical level, it is important to remember that:

> Vygotsky was not a bigoted intellectual who knew only his own discipline and pet hypothesis. On the contrary, he was a man of immense culture who kept abreast of the recent development in literature, drama, the fine arts, and music. Above all, Vygotsky absorbed the new theater performances and the new poems and novels. … He was also personally acquainted with the poets Mandel'shtam and Ehrenburg and the film director Eisenstein. He frequented Tairov's Chamber Theater and Meyerhold's and Stanislavsky's Art Theater. From about 1920 to 1923, he worked in Gomel as the local cultural official. In this capacity, he travelled all over Russia to bring the best theatrical companies to Gomel.
>
> *(Van der Veer, 2007, p. 24)*

Vygotsky's first great love was theatre. He wrote his first essay, *Tragedy of Hamlet Prince of Denmark* (1915), when he was nineteen, shortly after the play was performed in Moscow in Konstantin Stanislavsky and Gordon Craig's version. He included this essay, emended, in his doctoral thesis, *Psychology of Art* (1925a). Later, Vygotsky became interested in the phenomenon of acting with his essay

On the Problem of the Psychology of the Actor's Creative Work (1932a). Already in his doctoral thesis, Vygotsky saw art as a mediation, a cultural instrument capable of regulating and transforming complex emotional reactions. In his theorisation, art can be seen as a "tool regarding feelings" in the social context.

This point of view evokes the sense of the cultural-historical theory advanced by the psychologist. In synthesis, according to Vygotsky's perspective, all semiotic systems, with the signs they propose and the meanings they convey, work as mediators, as cultural instruments devised to produce, regulate, and transform complex reactions which encompass both emotions and reason. Through the mediation of signs, elementary psychological functions acquire a complex structure, becoming higher psychological functions. These are the highest *qualitatively human* processes, where both intellectual and emotional aspects are involved. In relation to the ways and context of this transformation, the specific human mental functioning is set in a necessarily cultural context.

The core of Vygotsky's cultural-historical theory can be brought out through a fundamental idea, according to which the overall historical evolution of human social and cultural activity interacts with the psychological development of individuals, determining the fundamental characteristics of their psychological functions. The Vygotskyan notion of culture is broad, and in general, it is the result of all the experience gained by humankind in deepening and making meaningful the world. Experiences and knowledge, collected and preserved, are embodied in psychological tools.

As Vygotsky wrote:

> Psychological tools are artificial formations. By their nature they are social and not organic or individual devices. They are directed toward the mastery of [mental] – one's or someone else's – just as technical devices are directed toward the mastery of processes of nature. The following may serve as examples of psychological tools and their complex systems: language, different forms of numeration and counting, mnemotechnic techniques, algebraic symbolism, works of art, writing, schemes, diagrams, maps, blueprints, all sorts of conventional signs.
>
> *(Vygotsky, 1930a; Engl. transl., p. 85)*

Art is a psychological medium, but it must be clarified that this idea of a tool is a complex concept which is not limited to signs and signalling systems. The nature of psychological tools cannot be reduced to their material existence. According to Vygotsky, psychological tools are to be recognised as practices embodied in human beings. Through them, the individuals transform themselves and transform the world around them, leaving a cultural legacy that is transferred from one generation to another. The Vygotskyan concept of a psychological tool becomes especially useful, as it will be illustrated, to orientate and understand the theoretical meaning of Eisenstein's ideas on art and especially film.

In the history of Soviet psychology, the period between 1925 and 1932 was particularly rich in ideas, both within the framework of Vygotsky's cultural-historical theory and within Luria's neuropsychological field of research. It was at that time that Eisenstein, close with both, developed an interest in the study of *methods* to be used in film research and, in a broader sense, in aesthetics.

This theme dominated the director's theoretical research from the early 1930s until his death. The ideas formulated on *method*, which is also the title of the rich and major collection of his writings on the subject, are linked to the cultural-historical paradigm. Eisenstein's aesthetic ideas, like the cultural-historical theory, imply the unity of psyche, brain, and sign systems that, for the filmmaker, represent the tools for artistic expression, including cinema.

At the same time, he shows interest in the mediated and indirect character of psychological processes and the general assumption of their historical quality. The main objective of the work *Metod* is to identify the fundamental rules of art, in all its forms, to apply them to both conceptual criticism and to the actual production of effective artistic works.

His early essays on montage had been influenced by a structuralist philosophical approach, linked to the ideas of Ferdinand de Saussure (1922) and tended to consider the single elements of films as complementary to the system, or rather to the *structure*. In *Metod*, written when he had reached a different maturity, the substantial characteristic of the approach adopted by the director is different, and it is presented by a determined and coherent historicism of Marxist extraction. In fact, in the name of dialectical philosophy, great attention is paid to the diachronic elements along with the evaluation of the synchronic aspects of reality.

Central to *Metod* is what he called the *Grundproblem*, the fundamental problem of art. The *Grundproblem* is the problem of the coexistence, in art, of the rational and the irrational, the conscious and the unconscious.

Eisenstein believes this coexistence is possible because, according to him, the human mind operates simultaneously on different evolutionary levels. Layers of logical thinking and layers of sensitive emotions coexist. Images in cinema and works of art, in general, must succeed in making these two layers work simultaneously.

It is a conception which echoes the Vygotskyan idea of "intelligent" emotions; in the socially organised human being, emotions must also be examined from the "cultural-historical" perspective. In this view, the aesthetic experience, successfully produced by a work of art, is conceived as a combination of a sensitive, emotional reaction and a rational understanding.

Eisenstein follows the idea of simultaneous functioning of different psychological levels, which is consistent with Vygotsky's perspective; following this path, he believes that the laws of artistic form are determined by the laws of so-called *sensual thinking* built on the inner patterns of human psychological functioning. Eisenstein defined this psychological functioning as archaic, pre-logical or magic.

To the director, sensual thinking represents, in the creation of the work of art, something more complex than what is pre-logical or the elements of the unconscious. Somehow, sensual thinking aims to contain all of them. As early as 1932, Otto Rank had emphasised the analogy between the terminology concerning Lévy-Bruhl's prelogical, Freud's terminology concerning the unconscious and Cassirer's terminology concerning myth (1923/1929). Eisenstein was familiar with these theoretical proposals.

One of the fundamental aspects of this perspective is that the psychological mechanisms the artists are supposed to activate to realise their work of art are the same the viewer uses to experience it. This is the thesis of isomorphism between creation and fruition, and between the two of them, art acts as an intermediary.

To follow this path, linked to the "Fundamental Problem", Eisenstein delves into the evolutionary sources of the psyche, looking for them – simultaneously – in the social and psychological evolution of the *homo sapiens* and in the biological evolution of life as such. In following this stream of thought, he faces the phenomenon of regression, in its various modes, and the desire for a "sinking into the mother's womb", notions which are embedded into psychoanalytical thought. The director's reflections on art and its manifestations, collected in *Metod*, are articulated in an anthropological and evolutionary perspective that progressively develops through several stages. As Somaini wrote in *Metod*

> Eisenstein formulates the idea according to which every emotionally powerful work of art bears in itself, in one way or another, the traces of early phases of biological, psychological or cultural history. Different "paths of regression" (*puti regressa*) are examined in the chapters of *Metod*, and all these "paths", according to Eisenstein, lead to some kind of synthetic, unified, undifferentiated state: "androgyny", reconsidered as a mystical unity of masculine and feminine that appearing in different ways in the history of philosophy, literature, and alchemy; "prelogical thinking", as a form of "diffused perception" characterized by the presence of what Lévy-Brühl had named "*loi de participation*", a belief in the magical interconnectedness of all beings; "protoplasmaticity", the state of all primitive organic forms which had not undergone any process of anatomic differentiation.
>
> *(Somaini, 2016, p. 44)*

In Eisenstein's theoretical perspective, this archaic and primordial "regressive force", translated into a historical dimension, generated "communism" as a social condition. In its primitive form, it preceded class division in archaic societies.

The idea of a biologically "archaic force" played a crucial role in Eisenstein's early ideas on montage. He was attracted to archaic phenomena and, due to the Pavlovian influence inherited from Meyerhold, the director aimed to study "not just men, but rather the 'primitive sociobiological' patterns. The film, in other words, was … a field for experiments, taking off from the simplest and most atavistic reflexes" (De Benedictis, 2001, p. 163). In the 1920s, the Pavlovian model, in its mechanistic simplicity, had addressed not only the new Russian generation of psychologists but, more generally, Russian culture. In art, the criterion of conditioned reflexes was used to achieve the highest emotional impact on the viewer. As Carroll aptly put it:

> The early Eisenstein held a very orthodox Pavlovian view of montage. Conflicting montage patterns, he believed, directly elicited unconditioned emotional responses: shocks of affect. In Eisenstein's view, this affect could be realized in the viewer as pathos … The proper stimuli elicit the proper response …
>
> *(Carroll, 1980, p. 22)*

Afterwards, the director's thought progressed towards the psychoanalytical model in its conceptual broadness, encompassing the paradigmatic dimension of the unconscious with its theoretical issues.

Eisenstein's later interest in Vygotsky and Luria's ideas represented a further maturation and development towards a more general and comprehensive theoretical framework, characterised by the complexity of the cultural-historical dimension wherein the individual psyche is connected to the social and historical environment in evolutionary terms.

The examination of anthropological, artistic, and cultural phenomena becomes important since through them, one can research cognitive life but, especially for Eisenstein, emotional life. At that stage, the director established a connection between the psychoanalytical dimension of the unconscious and the cultural-historical theory.

In the second part of *Metod*, we have several examples of this approach, drawn from some scenes extracted from Dostoevsky and Tolstoy, images of Dürer and Leonardo, Balinese rites and dances, some theatre settings of the Chinese director May Lai Fan, etc. In his speculations, the director goes far beyond the aesthetic or anthropological level. The "sinking into the mother's womb", the *Mutterliebe Versenkung*, or MLB, acquires a political connotation. As already said, the prenatal phase is compared to the period before the biologically most mature and current stage of the development of the human species. This comparison also extends to the social dimension, in its earliest forms, of the primitive societies prior to class division.

Since Eisenstein embraced the Vygotskyan idea that the individual psyche was the product of the historical, social, and cultural context, he investigated, psychologically, the "particular forms" of thinking and behaviour in that specific and archaic historical situation. Furthermore, the director seemed convinced that true art owned an internal and privileged connection to that original dimension, both on an individual and collective level.

Vygotsky was the first to pose the question of the historical development of humanity and its consequences on the individual psyche. Many ideas by Eisenstein, like the notion of inner monologue, which is developed for film, are related to Vygotsky's ideas, collected in *Thinking and Speech* (1934).

Vygotsky believes that the historical development of human beings is *qualitatively* different from that of animals. On a methodological level, regarding psychology, the overcoming of the "stimulus-response" model offered by Pavlov, following the footsteps of Bekhterev's work, is already implicit in this statement: "We might say that every basically new approach to scientific problems inevitably leads to new methods and ways of research" (Vygotsky, 1931; Engl. transl., p. 27).

Vygotsky looks for new methodological criteria for research and experimentation in the discipline of psychology. In his search for a methodology, he turned to Marxism and to Engels' ideas.

The Dialectics of Nature by Friedrich Engels (written in 1883 but never printed before) was published in Russia in 1925 and had a strong impact on the Soviet culture of the time. The presence of these Engelsian ideas, which Eisenstein also studied, is fundamental to Vygotsky.

It is beyond the scope of the present work to provide a detailed analysis of Engels' ideas, but we should note that Vygotsky's thought and Eisenstein's ideas are connected to the ideas expressed by Engels and to the Marxist heritage, including Lenin's concepts portrayed in *Materialism ed Empirio-Criticism* (1909).

More specifically, the already mentioned theory of reflection, or mirroring, assumes the objectivity of the external world and knowledge as reflection, first sensory and then extended to any form of knowledge; furthermore, the idea that the succession of one scientific theory to another does not depend on their conventionality, but on the greater insight into reality achieved by the new theories. Finally, the criterion of praxis is related to the importance of keeping a strong bond between theory and practice, which validates the theoretical results. Vygotskyan criteria for the method are connected to the philosophical concept of reflex, derived from Marxism. This reflex, which is different from the Pavlovian one, allows us to historicise and decline – culturally – the contents of psychological reality.

With concern to Engelsian theoretical proposals, Vygotsky stated that we must oppose naturalistic and mechanistic approaches, according to which it is only nature that acts on human beings and historical development is determined by natural conditions. In fact, the relationship must be seen as dialectical, and it must be borne in mind that human beings, in turn, act on nature.

The psychologist claims that this assumption must underpin any study and interpretation of higher psychological functions; the objective is to identify and adhere to a methodology that is philosophically materialist and suited to the demands of the new experimental psychology. Following this approach, Vygotsky proposes *three principles*:

I *Analysing processes, not things*. A distinction must be made between the analysis of a thing and that of a process. In a discipline such as psychology,

> the mental process itself, whether we speak of the development of speech or volition, is a process that undergoes certain changes before our eyes … If we replace analysis of things with analysis of process, then the basic problem for consideration becomes the genetic restoration of all the instances of development of

> the given process. Here, the principal task of analysis is restoring the process to its initial stage or, in other words, converting a thing into a process.
>
> *(Vygotsky, 1931; Engl. transl., p. 68)*

II *Explanation vs. description.* The psychological analysis must keep away from nominal descriptions and try to investigate the causal and dynamic relations of phenomena: "The real task of analysis in any science is specifically to disclose the real causal-dynamic relations and connections that lie at the base of any phenomena" (Vygotsky, 1931; Engl. transl., p. 68).

III *The problem of "solidified behaviour".*

> In psychology, we often are confronted with processes that have already become solidified, that is, passed through a very long historical development and were converted into a kind of fossil. Behavioral fossils most often are found in so-called automated or mechanical mental processes. These processes, which as a result of long functioning are perfected in the millionth repetition, become automatic and lose their initial appearance.
>
> *(Vygotsky, 1931; Engl. transl., p. 71)*

These fossilised processes are not remnant traces of biological evolution but

> residues of the historical development of behaviour: ... what must interest us is not the finished result, not the sum or product of development, but the very process of genesis or establishment of the higher form caught in a living aspect. For this, the researcher must very frequently transform the automatic, mechanical, fossilized character of the higher form and turn its historical development back, experimentally return the form that we are interested into its initial moments in order to make it possible to trace the process of its genesis. But as we have already said, this is what the problem of dynamic analysis involves.
>
> *(Vygotsky, 1931; Engl. transl., p. 71)*

Eisenstein embraced Vygotskyan's ideas, both in his interpretation of history and in the making of the artistic work. The Vygotskyan idea of higher stages of development dialectically and functionally connected to the past stimulated Eisenstein's artistic research, which saw in the arts the co-presence of regression and progress.

They both believed that the laws of dialectical materialism, understood as a method, could grasp the features of any object historically mutable that was *in motion.* This applied both to speech and art.

Eisenstein was interested both in the individual and the various forms of social expression because, adopting the dialectical method, individual history entered the scene, intertwining with the history of the species and the historical world.

Echoing Engels' terminology, Vygotsky often used the expression "dialectical leap". When the psychologist started to investigate mental phenomena in their unfolding, he studied their processes of transformation.

These transformations imply, philosophically, dialectical leaps. With his work, Vygotsky eventually outlined for his friend Eisenstein a methodology and a system of ideas that were firmly organised on a philosophical level. This firmness and conceptual depth are the basis of the major influence exerted by Vygotskyan thought, not only on contemporary figures such as Eisenstein but on the history of psychology and on a wide range of human disciplines. This influence on the psychological theoretical heritage and the world of culture, in general, took place especially from the second half of the twentieth century, the same period in which Vygotsky's ideas spread.

An in-depth examination of the philosophical basis of Vygotsky's ideas is beyond our scope, but it should be highlighted, as a founding concept, that his anti-dualistic perspective had Spinoza's theory as a basic reference point (Steila, 2007). Vygotsky praised the methodological criterion through which Spinoza approached the study of human feelings:

> In the argument between causal psychology and teleological psychology, in the argument between the deterministic and nondeterministic conceptions of feelings, in the confrontation between the spiritualistic and materialistic hypotheses, Spinoza must be placed on the side of those who defend the scientific conception of human feelings against the metaphysical.
>
> *(Vygotsky, 1931–1933; Engl. transl., p. 221)*

Add to this the affirmation of a material constitution of the human psyche and the fight against the confusion between the gnoseological and ontological planes.

This last trait echoed Lenin's mentioned epistemologically founded struggle against Empirio-Criticism and the thought of Mach and Avenarius. On the gnoseological level, according to classical philosophy, the psyche is autonomous in its cognitive function and confronts the external world, matter, and body. Faced with knowledge, the subject abstracts itself from its body detaches itself from it and explores it as if it were a foreign object.

This distinction must not be transferred to the ontological level, as if the psyche and body were two separate entities. This division also takes place with respect to the psyche itself. The cognitive psyche, the ego, sets its own psyche, thoughts, and memories as its object. The confusion between the gnoseological and ontological levels had been typical of the so-called Machists, opposed by Lenin.

Vygotsky's critical examination of all his contemporary schools of psychology conducted in *The Historical Meaning of the Crisis in Psychology* (1927) is very important. This work represents a premise for Vygotsky to introduce a new, non-absolutist theoretical model consistent with the methodological indications coming from the Marxist and Engelsian dialectics. This non-abstract model sets the material dimension of the mind within its historical origins, suggesting an original solution to that dualist opposition inherited from Descartes, which still looms heavily on psychology, psychoanalysis, and the so-called human sciences.

Furthermore, this line of thought offers very new theoretical tools for evaluating social products and activities. Art, certainly, is a central objective within this discourse.

As mentioned, Vygotsky defined the idea of a gradual and linear evolutionary psychological process naïf. According to dialectical philosophy, a real transformation implies a "leap", a qualitative acquisition of new properties.

This approach has important and original outcomes, especially in the psychological development of the child. Dialectically, this development is characterised by periodicity, irregularity in the emergence of distinct functions and the qualitative transformation of one form into another. Thanks to this idea, Vygotsky outlined a new model of the functioning of the psyche and individual history. Evolution and revolution do not come one after the other; they belong to each other, in a qualitative relationship that progresses, precisely, through dialectical leaps; "In Hegel's view, the dialectical qualifies that which – while retaining the initial elements – has acquired *new* properties" (Mecacci, 2017, p. 41).

The same perspective, in a different field, gradually penetrated Eisenstein's thought. In the words of Bordwell:

> In 1929 Eisenstein begins to frame questions of form of film and effect in dialectical terms ... He starts from the Engels-Lenin view that every phenomenon, natural or social, constitutes a tense field of opposed forces pressing towards a synthesis, at a higher level ... The individual artwork is also a dialectical whole ... He also posits a dialectical epistemology, whereby the very process of coming to know reflects the actual course of the world. That is, correct thinking is dialectical in form. For Eisenstein, who always treats form as a process, the agitational artwork must not only reflect the dynamic of the world but also provoke the spectator into patterns of thought. Intellectual cinema has a new task; it will teach the worker to think dialectically. Eisenstein proceeds to recast his conception of film form in terms of dialectical conflict.
>
> *(Bordwell, 1993, pp. 128–130)*

The director places the laws of dialectical materialism at the basis of his ideas; philosophically, Eisenstein wants *a universal method to understand phenomena in motion and in a reciprocal relation to each other*. This is true for the psyche and for cinema.

On a historical level, Eisenstein drew inspiration from Vygotsky's thought. This is reflected in many contexts, and it was officially announced in the speech he gave at the Soviet Film Workers' Conference in 1935. In his talk, the director refers directly to the experimental psychology of Vygotsky and Luria as a way to pose "new problems" to the cinema.

In 1934, Vygotsky had investigated the issue of methodology in the opening of his fundamental work *Thinking and Speech* (1934).

The psychologist focuses on speech because it is in the word that the property of meaning lies. *Meaning* lies in the *inner part* of the word and defines the relation between thinking and speech. Meaning is the core of a unity called "verbal thought" and, mostly, does not refer to a single object but to a whole group or class of objects. Meaning is a *generalisation*, "[it] is a *verbal act of thought*; its reflection of reality differs radically from that of immediate sensation or perception" (Vygotsky, 1934; Engl. transl., p. 45).

In the Engelsian idea of "dialectical leaps", the first leap is from non-thinking matter to sensation. However, there is also a qualitatively different leap in the passage from immediate sensation to thought. Thought can reflect reality in a *generalised* way; in fact, higher psychological functions specific to human beings are possible because of the ability to reflect reality in a generalised manner. Furthermore, the fundamental human capability to develop social relationships depends on this capability to generalise. Social relations are made possible by rational understanding and by intentional transmission of both thought and lived experience mediated by language. Dialectically, speech is "a system that emerged with the need to interact socially in the labour process" (Vygotsky, 1934; Engl. transl., p. 46).

The hint to human work implies a connection with the work of Marx and Engels. Connecting with Engels, welcoming "the influence of nature on man", Vygotsky claims that man acts on nature and determines new natural conditions of existence. Art, for Vygotsky, is part of this human action in the natural world. To fully outline the aspects of Vygotsky's thought that most attracted Eisenstein, it is useful to refer to the concept of the "psychological tool".

It is important to underline that the meaning of Vygotsky's work refers to culture and, above all, to the way the individual – at the developmental stage – appropriates and internalises it. There is no direct relationship between the subject and culture in terms of an abstract entity. The relationship is indirect, mediated by other people or by *tools* that these same people provide to the child and that are acquired during the developmental phase. This mediation is not simply a human relationship between child and adult, but to be implemented, it *requires*, a set of specific tools.

The notion of the tool is central to Vygotsky's work. The same topic was also a subject of interest in psychology for Wolfgang Köhler (1917), an exponent of Gestalt psychology. Examining the subject, Vygotsky observed that human beings inherit the use of tools, unlike animals. Each generation has tools that change and are renewed in the course of human history; new tools appear over time. Moreover, animals do not possess an elaborate speech that enables them to communicate on the use of these tools.

In human beings, according to Vygotsky, speech itself is a psychological tool which communicates and provides information on the use of any potentially available tool. This is a founding concept; speech is an external tool that the psyche encounters and acquires in its development.

Finally, in the Marxist perspective adopted by both Vygotsky and Eisenstein, the use of tools plays a fundamental role in work, i.e., the social organisation, which is absent in the animal world, which allows humanity to adapt to the environment. This concept echoes Engels' ideas: the production and use of tools constitute not only the hallmark of the human species but also the pivot of historical evolution.

In the years before Vygotsky's work began to circulate, Russian reflexology, with Pavlov and Bekhterev, based all human behaviour and reactions on the stimulus-response mechanism drawn from observation and experimentation on the animal world. In the human species, however, we can observe different mental situations. In human beings, it is possible to generate new responses by virtue of independent processes that are not automatically linked to the stimulus-response process. These are mental processes. In Marxist philosophical terms, of Hegelian derivation, they take place on an "ideal" level. Practically, the translation of these processes means that a bee building the hive by virtue of a set of responses, or innate species-specific reactions, is qualitatively different, in the way it works, from an architect. The architect, to paraphrase Marx (1867; Engl. transl., vol. 1, Part 3, p. 178), builds the work first in his own head, differently from the bee; the result exists in the mind of the architect before work begins.

From a wider historical perspective, the notion of tool has impacted different moments in the history of philosophical thought. Looking back, Bacon and Spinoza – authors who were appreciated and cited by Vygotsky and Luria – had outlined a difference between the "tools of the hand" and the "tools of the mind" (see Mecacci, 2017, p. 47). Following this line of thought, Vygotsky distinguishes between "material tools", concerning the activity carried out by human beings in the external world, and "psychological tools", related to the activity carried out within the mind. The "material tools" are instruments in the common sense of the term, such as the hammer, the fork, the pen, or, nowadays, the camera and the computer. They help us do things that are not possible with the use of our hands. Nevertheless, their use depends on knowledge and plans that are internal to the mind. Both the tools and the knowledge related to them are historically generated and passed on from one generation to the other. Material tools are related to the human activity carried out in the external world, while "psychological tools" concern the activity carried out within the mind. According to Vygotsky, this division is not to be intended in a mechanical way but in a philosophically dialectical way.

Psychological tools are the most complex systems of the human mind. Mecacci highlights that "while material tools related to the activity of human beings act in the *external* world, psychological tools relate to the activity performed *inside* the mind itself" (Mecacci, 2017, pp. 47, 48). According to Vygotsky, language, computation, writing, and artworks are examples of these tools and their complex systems.

Art is a psychological tool for the concreteness of the artistic products. The instruments of psychological mediation play a role both in processes within the individual mind and in processes between one mind and another. Vygotsky defines "artificial" the tools that have been "invented" for different uses at a particular moment in human (historical) evolution. They have, therefore, a historical and social origin but impact on the psychological activity of the individual for several reasons.

The concept of the *tool* in cinema should be understood primarily as a technological acquisition and, at the same time, as a *mental instrument* capable of opening new communicative possibilities. From a historical perspective,

> cinema and photography, even before, could develop thanks to that substratum of technical knowledge that, especially with regards to chemistry and mechanics, received a great impulse from the necessities of industrial production between the end of the eighteenth century and the first half of the nineteenth century.
>
> *(Angelini, 1983, p. 29)*

Tools which are concrete and exist physically produce new mental situations. The clearest example is written signs, but cinema too can be considered an instrument of artificial psychological mediation. It is connected to a technological material reality and can also offer artistic production and communication, given specific conditions. Throughout the twentieth century, cinema was an expressive and communicative tool that, together with television, polarised the interests and emotions of the masses. The third millennium is dominated by computers, and the expressive potentials of this new tool are still under scrutiny and exploration.

As Mecacci stated

> [t]o use a given psychological tool, a particular organisation of the human mind is necessary, which differs from the organisation prior to the introduction of the new tool. This implies a rearrangement of pre-existing psychological functions, in parallel with a rearrangement of the related brain functions.
>
> *(Mecacci, 2017, p. 48)*

These rearrangements have a social origin and may continue, to different degrees, throughout the individual's life. They are based on a psychological 'toolkit' that is acquired by the individuals in their psychological development and within a certain historical-cultural context.

Shifting to cinema, these concepts open an interpretative window into the evolution of film language and its interaction with the social environment. Noticeably, to be understood by the spectators, a film must propose a language and, consequently, a montage that is consistent with the historical-cultural context in which the film is conceived and made. Any language, including film language, is structured and changes according to historical and cultural changes in society. Cinema language has undergone many changes from its origins to the present day. The enhancement in the choice of shots and angles, which has enriched the history of early cinema, is not only an autonomous improvement of the film medium but should also be related to the overall development of the social world in which cinema is placed and in which many authors have worked.

Eisenstein delved into this concept, drawing examples from the history of art. A noble example of this is the pictorial perspective introduced after feudalism, at a time when changes in the social context prepared and activated new perceptive differentiations in the psychological process of visual perception. As regards cinema, the changes that have occurred in recent years in the criteria and rhythms of film editing and in productions aimed to entertain assume, in the light of these concepts, a meaning connected to the demands of the social and productive world.

Eisenstein gives many significant examples of how framing and montage transfer meanings. Particularly interesting is the analysis of the so-called "pars pro toto" mechanism, which represents a phenomenon of symbolisation in montage. The director uses his own film, *Battleship Potemkin*, as an example; the scene in which the pince-nez glasses of the ship's doctor, framed in a close-up, synecdochically, represent the whole character. This process of symbolisation, which on a literary level can be compared to the rhetorical figure known as "synecdoche", also belongs, according to the director, to the criteria of inner language and primitive thought. It is what happens, for example, when a primitive man, adorning himself with the tooth of a killed animal, imagines he is carrying the equivalent of the whole animal.

In this analysis of the psychological meanings of cinema, it is of paramount importance to highlight the historical context in which the phenomenon takes place. This is because *living historical context transforms the criteria employed to conceive shots, the method to be used in filming and montage, and the viewer's perceptive abilities*.

With concern to this aspect of the cinematic language, which is always in progress, it is useful to make an example. The use of a "hand-held camera", held by the operator and not set on the tripod or fixed support, was the object of speculation.

In the past, image stabilisation – which is today achieved electronically – was a fantasy, a daring desire, a tale about the future. In fact, the use of hand-held cameras produced jolting images, and for the spectator, it was quite annoying. For most of the twentieth century, the idea to avoid at the utmost its use was accepted and shared by most cinema authors. Exceptions were made for specific cases. In general, besides rare situations linked to specific script needs, the hand-held camera was for very intense action scenes, like war films, thrillers, and the like.

At the end of the last century, the *Dogma 95 film movement*, born in Denmark with the aim to "purify" cinema from the "gangrene" of special effects and billion-dollar investments, introduced the hand-held camera as a characterising and frequent tool. Since then, films and TV productions began to use this technique again, becoming a sort of filmic "linguistic quirk" and, for a luckily brief period, an almost compulsory feature. The effects were, in some cases, paradoxical with aesthetic results, which must be debated and contextualised to the point that, nowadays, there is a tendency towards a return to a classic film language. Furthermore, the progress in shooting techniques helped to animate, with a hand-held camera, action scenes, keeping the movement but avoiding jolts.

Moreover, focusing the attention on simultaneous changes in the perceptive abilities of the average spectator, one should evaluate the transformations in reception tools. There has been a passage from cinema to TV screens and nowadays, videos are made and can be seen from smartphones, tablets and computers. The naïf language, used by the mass public in audio-visual communication, in their private life and their social media, had brought to an acceptance, in cinema montage, of attacks between sequences that were previously considered blatant errors.

A useful example is given by "overrun", that directors usually tend to avoid but when it happens, it is now perceived only by a "cinematically finely educated public". This is because overruns are done continuously in videos taken with cell phones and on social media.

The psychological tool of film language, which manifests primarily in montage, changes with historical and social conditions. The higher psychological functions dialectically change both in the perceptive dimension and, of course, in the conceptual dimension. Luria (1962) examined the transformation of cortical functions in relation to changes in psychological function.

Regarding the complex concept of the tool, it is important to remember that it can be an external tool, like a notebook, a computer, or a camera but it can also be inner, like a technique to memorise things or, above all, like the speech. Speech plays the most significant role in organising the human mind. It is an instrument of communication and, as Vygotsky claimed, an instrument of thought. In this perspective, film technology is an external tool and montage, as a mental operation, is an inner tool and a specific language.

In Eisenstein's thought, the issue of language is crucial; his ideas on "inner monologue" are connected, by analogy, to Vygotskyan concepts of "inner speech". For Vygotsky, the use of tools, together with the use of signs, can be near to the broader concept of "mediation activity". He highlighted that the notion of mediation was already present in Hegel (see Mecacci, 2017, p. 50). Hegel considered mediation the most typical activity of reason. Marx further developed this Hegelian concept. Marx extended it, in a philosophically materialistic sense, to work tools. Conceptually, Vygotsky completed the picture with an analysis of the use of signs.

Eisenstein's statements on the absolute technological and expressive novelty represented by the cinema in the social context are in tune with the concept of the medium outlined above. The film director, who came from theatre and found the theatrical dimension expressively insufficient, was conscious of the innovative strength of the film medium and eventually believed that it could surpass theatre.

When he first got in contact with cinema, Eisenstein felt the power that one feels seeing a tool that makes its first appearance in history, as with any other technological means, as the result of advances in human work and technology. Moreover, he perceived the revolutionary potential of the new medium not only in an artistic sense. According to him, cinema was destined to give life to "the construction of that new region of culture that will have to take the place of theatre" (*On the Didactic Program of the Proletkult Theatre Workshops*, in Eisenstein, 1998, Ital. transl., p. 235).

In line with these words, a couple of years later, the director switched completely to cinema, beginning to work on his first feature film, *Strike*, released in 1925. Embracing cinema, an innovative tool and expressive medium still to develop, Eisenstein quickly rejected the traditional idea of art. He questioned aesthetic formalism and naturalism, aiming to achieve an art capable of merging with the activity of the means of production and social life. Formalism, as an aesthetic current, had initially attracted the attention of Vygotsky himself. As Wertsch wrote:

> The Formalists argued that in order to study "literariness," one must identify and examine the linguistic devices and principles that characterize it ... Formalists' insistence on studying objective linguistic facts was consistent with Vygotsky's desire to outline an objective science of human mental functioning.
>
> *(Wertsch, 1985, pp. 82, 83)*

The idea of an industrial art capable of taking over the mechanical processes of production and of appropriating the new tools offered by technology, was spreading. This atmosphere of longing for progress characterised the entire Soviet society, which, in those years, in the economic sphere, was expressed in the NEP (New Economic Policy). In the field of economy, between 1921 and 1929, the NEP gave life to a measured liberalisation in production and trade.

Like other filmmakers at the beginning of the last century, with passion and amazement, Eisenstein ventured into this new land offered by emerging film technology. In 1934, he wrote:

> In the early 1920s we all came to the Soviet cinema as something not yet existent. We came upon no ready-built city; there were no squares, no streets laid out; not even little crooked lanes and blind alleys, such as we may find in the cinemetropolis of our day. We came like bedouins or goldseekers to a place with unimaginably great possibilities, only a small section of which has even now been developed. We pitched our tents and dragged into camp our experiences in varied fields. Private activities, accidental past professions, unguessed crafts, unsuspected eruditions-all were pooled and went into the building of something that had, as yet, no written traditions, no exact stylistic requirements, nor even formulated demands.
>
> *(Eisenstein, 1934, Through Theatre to Film; in: Eisenstein, 1949, p. 5., 1964, p. 5)*

Eisenstein's psychological knowledge profoundly influenced his approach to cinema-making. In his writings, he expressed the need to give a specific conceptual characterisation to montage.

On the one hand, cinema is articulated in its material technological concreteness, and on the other, in a process that requires montage as a psychological instrument, a mental operation, with its specific filmic language. Montage is the new psychological instrument that comes to life dialectically from the new technological tool. Montage is, first of all, an *instrument of communication*, a language whose characteristics contribute, connecting with it, to the social formation of the mind. Vygotsky's general directions on inner psychological tools also apply to montage:

> If the primary function of psychological tools such as language is to communicate, it is reasonable to expect these mediational means to be formed in accordance with the demands of communication. If these means also play an important role in shaping individuals' mental processes, we can expect such processes to be indirectly shaped by forces that originate in the dynamics of communication.
>
> *(Wertsch, 1985, p. 81)*

Since his first work, *Strike*, completed at the end of 1924, Eisenstein had used the innovation of an original and extreme use of montage in a psychological sense;

> Everyone who has had in his hands a piece of film to be edited knows by experience how neutral it remains, even though a part of a planned sequence, until it is joined with another piece, when it suddenly acquires and conveys a sharper and quite different meaning than that planned for it at the time of filming.
>
> *(Eisenstein, 1949, p. 10)*

Beyond the specific declinations which montage undertook in Eisenstein's work, "montage of attractions, intellectual and vertical", Eisenstein's general idea of montage has its own overall and characteristic conceptual value. Montage starts from an undifferentiated datum and then proceeds to a decomposition and subsequent differentiation. Subsequently, the elements are recomposed, and the initial datum is reproposed in a generalised manner and at a qualitatively higher level in a philosophical sense. This operation, in its simple nature, is found in all artistic forms, from writing to painting, from ancient to contemporary techniques. The practice of montage consists of the double work of decomposition and reassembling. To re-propose "at a higher level" means to restore the datum in an artistic manner, according to an organisation that contains the individual parts in a whole, offering a new sense which can be generalised. In this way, the datum moves away, for Eisenstein, from simple evidence and is invested with a universally communicable meaning;

> For us the microcosm of montage had to be intended like a unity that, in the intimate tension of contradictions, breaks to be then reassembled in a new unity

> on a new level, qualitatively superior, with images perceived in a new way … Montage became for us the means to achieve a unity of a superior order, the means to have, through montage of figurative concepts, the organic embodiment of a single idea, capable to embrace all the elements, the details, the parts of the film … We are reaching the moment in which – not only through montage but also through the synthesis of the idea, the drama of the actor, sound, tridimensionality and coloured cinematic representation – that same great rule of unity and diversity which is at the basis of our philosophy and that invests the whole montage methodology … will be transformed in the unity of the whole scheme on the level of conceptual figuration.
>
> *(Eisenstein, 2002; Ital. transl., vol. 2, p. 174)*

In this perspective, montage becomes the main instrument of the process or "living drama" of thought in the Vygotskyan sense; therefore, drama retains the meaning of the Greek word, which is to say, it expresses an *action*. It is a philosophically dialectical action which produces a synthesis between primitive emotions, "living remnants of ancient epochs" still active in civilisation and "the structure of the higher form" (Vygotsky, 1931; Engl. transl., p. 70). The term "drama" was used by the French psychologist George Politzer, founder, in 1929 of the *Revue de Psychologie Concréte*. The aim was to suggest an alternative vision of psychology, different from the academic one, considered distant from the psychological problems people generally face. The Marxist perspective did not intend to pay attention to an abstract being but to real people interacting and living in a cultural and social context.

For Vygotsky, the concept of "living drama" comes from a re-elaboration of the materialistic dialectical idea. Therefore, it is principally historical. Thinking and speech meet in human history. All the psychological theories which separate conscience from reality are to be criticised:

> These perspectives share a common point that is inherent to nearly all theories of thinking and speech. They share a profound and fundamental antihistorical perspective. All these theories oscillate between the poles of pure naturalism and pure spiritualism. They view thinking and speech in isolation from their history. However, only *an historical psychology, only an historical theory of inner speech, has the capacity to lead us to a correct understanding of this complex and extraordinary problem* … The relationship of thought to word is a vital process that involves the birth of thought in the word. Deprived of thought, the word is dead.
>
> *(Vygotsky, 1934; Engl. transl., p. 284)*

We can thus understand the impact Vygotsky's work had in the formulation of "inner monologue" for Eisenstein. Psychology, like any other human discipline, was, for Eisenstein, an opportunity to investigate the individual in general and, above all, to look at the human being as a producer of images and, thus, of art. Film montage, in the idea of the director, had to go from physical movement to more complex forms of mental movement, where metaphorical comparisons prevail over conceptual ones. The dialectical dimension manifests also in the relation between the director's mind and the film. In fact, dialectically, on the one hand, cinema must be built according to the same laws that regulate the material world to be organic; it must reproduce, with formal means, the process of growth and transformation that characterises living organisms. On the other hand, the same cinematic art, being the work and creation of a person, acts on her/him according to a simultaneous double movement. Films start from a datum of the real world, but its composition is a work of the director's mind that makes it beyond the data of concrete reality.

It is the laws of dialectics that allow the director to consider work as a synthetical and organic unity, connecting the evolutive process of the artistic product to the natural one – of living beings – and the historical one of societies. Technically speaking, it makes this theoretical hypothesis possible.

Eisenstein is also conscious that the psychological instrument of montage is destined to change, in a parallel way, with the technological changes of cinema tools. His ideas on the complex effects of montage, due to the advent of sound and colour in cinema, testify to this consciousness. Also, in this case, the theoretical framework comes from Vygotsky. He stated that "artificial tools", so-called because "invented" in a certain moment of historical development, in order to be used needed a particular organisation of the human mind, different to the one existing before the introduction of the new tool itself. It is a situation in which the theory on the ZPD finds expression; "… a psychological function appears twice: first on the social plane, and then on the psychological level. As a consequence, to put it in current terminology, psychological functions are basically "socially distributed"" (Haenen, Schrijnemakers and Stufkens, 2003, p. 251). This entails a re-restructuring of pre-existing psychological functions, which is parallel to a re-structuration of the relative brain functions. As already mentioned, Luria, who welcomed Vygotsky's ideas, devoted most of his activity to this kind of neuropsychological research (see Luria, 1962).

During the last century, cinema technology has significantly changed. We should not think only about sound and colour but also about the transformations that Eisenstein could only fantasise about, and that became a reality, like the use of IT and electronics for cinematic purposes.

Eisenstein's intuitions anticipated great technical changes but, above all, the transformation of the filmic language, which went through the twentieth century and continues today. The director was extremely interested in technological innovations. The attention paid to the introduction of sound revealed that interest, for example, in the declaration on *A Statement on Sound* signed in 1928 with Vsevolod Pudovkin and Grigorij Aleksandrov. In this declaration, they talk about the risk – that never happened – that the "talkie" could be invaded by theatre, regressing to a theatrical visual dimension. This did not happen because the image is, perceptively and cognitively, more "powerful" than words. Moreover, and fundamentally, for the theatrical situation to become effective, it is necessary for the relationship between actor and public to exist in a real living dimension. Film and TV footage, when they are visualised, have a different emotional intensity and effectiveness compared to live performances (see Angelini, 2014, p. 20). In a broader sense, cinema can evoke extraordinarily strong emotions because it possesses *a trait of reality*, while theatre, even if it is never *fake*, is *false*, and the public is happy to be part of this fiction. Eisenstein, who came from theatre, proposed different ideas on cinema specificity.

It is useful to point out that the psychological differences in the perception of cinema compared to theatre depend mostly on the phenomenon of "projective identification" that shall be further illustrated.

Eisenstein, Pudovkin, and Aleksandrov feared that the specific peculiarity of cinema, with the introduction of sound, could be influenced by theatre. In *A Statement of Sound* (1928), they outline solutions to avoid this risk. Besides the credibility of the fears expressed in the declaration, it is an important document because it testifies to the awareness that cinema is everchanging. This change takes place both concretely, in a technological sense – and subjectively, in relation to the author's elaboration and the viewer's psychological reception. Eisenstein, strongly committed to art issues, questioned how the psychological organisation, imposed on the spectator by the innovative technologies, could have modified the artistic perception. Moreover, in the conclusion of *A Statement of Sound* (1928), it is suggested that the new tool of sound could resolve several expressive problems that the technical limitations of silent cinema had to face.

On several occasions, the director talked about colour, especially in the period between 1946 and 1948. Colour is considered one of the formal aspects of *synaesthesia* (see Cervini, 2006, p. 87) that contributes to the filmmaking. Colour can be one of the elements that determine, with its appearance, the psychological reorganisation of the spectator's mind.

Eisenstein advanced the idea that the problem of montage, in all its expressive aspects, was a psychological issue. Initially, investigating the topic, he referred to the notion of "inner speech", and then – talking about the description of the mental work necessary for the realisation of montage – he used the term "inner monologue", also hinting at the psychology of language elaborated by Vygotsky.

We must remember that the methodological approach of the psychologist to speech was systemic. He considered thinking and speech two inter-functional evolutive lines that could not be studied separately. Splitting thinking from speech, as happened in some fields of traditional linguistics and psychology, was a mistake according to Vygotsky, or rather, it represented a spiritualist approach contrary to history. For the psychologist, it was important to approach this scientific problem in a new way;

> For this reason, research acquires a completely different form and course when it is linked to finding a new method suitable to the new problem; in that case, it

> differs radically from those forms in which the study simply applies developed and established scientific methods to new areas.
>
> *(Vygotsky, 1931; Engl. transl., p. 44)*

Vygotsky was interested in the new research, contemporary to him, like that of de Saussure, which emphasised the strong bond between sound and meaning in words. He delved into Piaget's thought through a complex confrontation, and in 1932 he wrote the Russian introduction to *Le language et la pensée* of the Swiss psychologist. In that period, Vygotsky was close to psychoanalytical thought, and in this introduction of about 60 pages, Freud and psychoanalysis are quoted 14 times. Although it is not substantial here to delve into the relationship between Piaget and Vygotsky, Yarosevsky wrote:

> Of all twentieth-century psychologists, probably only Piaget can be compared to him. But unlike Vygotsky, Piaget did not study the problems associated with art and literature, and even though he had studied biology, he did not conduct research in neurology, defectology, or psychiatry.
>
> *(Yarosevsky, 1996, p. 168)*

In a context related to images, though, it is interesting to remember that Piaget made some hypotheses on visual thought while dealing with autistic thought:

> Autistic thought is subconscious …it creates for itself a dream world of imagination; it tends, not to establish truths, but to satisfy desires, and it remains strictly individual and incommunicable as such by means of language. On the contrary, it works chiefly by images, and in order to express itself, has recourse to indirect methods, evoking by means of symbols and myths the feeling by which it is led … autism undoubtedly calls into being and enrich many inventions which are subsequently clarified and demonstrated by intelligence … Directed thought, as it develops, is controlled more and more by the laws of experience and of logic in the stricter sense. Autistic thought, on the contrary, obeys a whole system of special laws (laws of symbolism and of immediate satisfaction) … Now these two forms of thought, whose characteristics diverge so profoundly, differ chiefly as to their origin, the one being socialized and guided by the increasing adaptation of individuals one to another, whereas the other remains individual and uncommunicated. Furthermore - and this is of the very first importance for the understanding of child thought – this divergence is due in large part to the following fact. Intelligence, just because it undergoes a gradual process of socialization, is enabled through the bond established by language between thoughts and words to make an increasing use of concepts; whereas autism, just because it remains individual, is still tied to images, to organic activity, and even to organic movements.
>
> *(Piaget, 1923; Engl. transl., pp. 43–45)*

Piaget believed that between these two opposite forms of thinking, a private and not communicable one (autistic thinking) and the other social and communicable (intelligent thinking or – as Vygotsky called it – logical thinking), there were in-between forms, the main one being "egocentric thinking".

This concept also emerges from Vygotsky's theory but with another meaning and other assumptions. Vygotsky outlines a theoretical reflection on the genesis of speech and its relationship to thought. *Speech is conceived as something that is external to the subject. In this perspective, language does not exist in the abstract and it is a product of thinking; it is already present in human culture and society when individuals are born and – with their brain – enter human history. Speech differs, just as societies differ, in relation to times, geographies, acquired customs, etc.*

The relation between thinking and speech is not to be interpreted as an "original link", but it is to be conceived as the result of a process that is both ontogenetic and phylogenetic. As mentioned, Vygotsky highlighted that, in the social world, speech existed before the development of thinking in the individual. It manifests in the child when thinking and language – which socially exist before thinking – meet and integrate. Through development they become structurally interdependent. In perspective, the entire formation of higher psychological functions is made possible by the internalisation of speech from the outside to the inside. This is a fundamental evolutionary passage. The child is conceived as a part of the social whole, like a subject of social relations who participates, from his earliest days, in collective life. The social is interpreted as something intrinsic and inseparable by the child, as a force that becomes its own, mentally, in childhood life.

Thinking and speech, two separate processes, integrate during individual development into a new unity which is meaning. Meaning, which connects a thought to a word, is changeable because it evolves with the historical and cultural development of the individual. Gradually, through parental and social relationships, external speech, which is present in society, enters the child's mind. According to Vygotsky, at around the age of three, interpersonal speech differentiates into a socialised language, with a communicative function towards others, and an *egocentric speech*, where the child speaks to herself/himself, to guide her/his thinking, solve problems and plan her/his actions.

Egocentric *speech* has its own organising function and later develops without ever disappearing. Egocentric speech evolves in *speech* as well. Furthermore, inner *speech*

> is not speech minus sound but a speech function that is unique in its structure and function. Correspondingly, it has an entirely different organization than external speech. It has its own syntax. One characteristic of egocentric speech that manifests a clear development tendency is its fragmentation and abbreviation.
>
> *(Vygotsky, 1934; Engl. transl., p. 266).*

In this process, the norms of cultural and speech acquisition are not natural laws but "historical and social".

Growing up, children refine their communication skills in their socialised verbal behaviour and modify and internalise the egocentric language in a progressive way until it becomes their own *inner speech*. Egocentric language relates to inner speech.

In fact, on the ontogenetic level, the progression in speech development is the same in Vygotsky and Piaget. The passage is from *autistic, non-verbal thinking* to *egocentric speech* and *egocentric thinking* and from the latter to *socialised speech* and *logical thinking*. However, for Piaget, the child goes from an initial stage of closed thinking to a final stage of thinking open to others and, therefore communicable. On the contrary, according to Vygotsky, the passage is from an initial stage of socialised thinking/speech to a final stage of inner thinking/speech.

The different opinions between the two scholars emerge in several contexts (see Haenen, Schrijnemakers, Stufkens, 2003, p. 251). According to Piaget, the child's egocentric speech disappears throughout development, morphing into social language. In contrast, for Vygotsky, the child's mind is socialised by speech; the stimulus of speech comes from outside; and the development of egocentric speech represents a developmental prerequisite for behavioural planning. In Vygotsky's perspective, egocentric speech never disappears but becomes an instrument of thinking that is latently present in the mental dynamics as a silent form of external *speech*.

Talking about the dispute between Vygotsky and Piaget, Etkind (see 1993, Chapter 5) suggests an original perspective, claiming that they were both profoundly influenced by the work of Sabina Spielrein, who, for some time, had studied child psychology from a psychoanalytical perspective;

> The year 1921 was crucial for twenty-five-year-old Jean Piaget. His cognitive energy, which had until then raced back and forth from the classification of mollusks to philosophical epistemology, finally found its focus. It was in 1921 that Piaget published his first article, devoted to children's speech and thought. Also in 1921, Piaget underwent psychoanalysis with Sabina Spielrein … A year before she met Piaget, in 1920, Sabina Spielrein "of Lausanne" presented a paper at the Sixth International Psychoanalytic Congress in The Hague. An abridged version was published in the official journal of the International Association under the title *On the Origin and Development of Speech*. Spielrein explained to her colleagues that there are two types of speech: autistic, which was not designed for communication, and social speech. Autistic speech was primal and served as the basis of social speech.
>
> *(Etkind, 1993, pp. 162, 163)*

Spielrein's influence was also important in relation to Vygotsky. At the Psychoanalytic Institute,

> Spielrein gave a course on the psychology of unconscious … Young Luria, the secretary of the Institute, and young Vygotsky … might well have attended

> her course, perceiving her lectures as the last word in international science … It seems likely that Spielrein served as a mediator between the two schools of world psychology, Jean Piaget's genetic psychology and Lev Vygotsky's cultural-historical psychology.
>
> *(Etkind, 1993, p. 173, 174)*

Studying the child's communication with parents, Vygotsky highlighted the emotional factors that Piaget tended to underestimate. Furthermore, Vygotsky always placed his psychological considerations within the philosophical framework of Marxism and, in the first phase of his studies, was remarkably close to psychoanalysis. This was a position shared by many intellectuals of the period, Eisenstein included. In December 1924, the psychologist gave a lecture at the Moscow Psychoanalytic Society on "The Use of the Psychoanalytic Method in Literature" (see *Internationale Zeitschrift für Psychoanalyse*, 2/1924, p. 136), and Sabina Spielrein was among the Muscovite members of the Society. On the relationship between Spielrein, Piaget and Vygotsky, Cooper-White and Brock Kelcourse (2019, p. 156) recently wrote that the Swiss scholar had carried out a psychoanalytical treatment with Spielrein for about eight months. Furthermore, Wilson and Weinstein (1992, 1996) have conducted a psychoanalytical reading of Vygotsky's ideas from a clinical perspective.

The closeness of inner speech and egocentric speech that, for Vygotsky, was typical of childhood attracted Eisenstein's interest. In the development of his ideas, he concluded that inner speech could be used in the artistic process and film. Following Eisenstein's ideas, inner speech shows certain characteristics that belong to sensual thinking, in particular, drive and emotional aspects. Affectivity represents a founding element of linguistic content (see Vygotsky, 1931–1933). It is important to remember that "sensual" inner speech is neither alternative nor secondary to logical speech. Inner speech is firmly established in the psyche in a way that is not only complementary to conceptual speech but also an essential vehicle of affective and volitional elements. For Vygotsky, it represented one of the different and interactive levels of the individual's verbal instrument, considered as a whole.

Furthermore, Vygotsky analysed the complex integration of thinking and speech on a semantic level in the context of meaning. It is worth remembering that the correlation between thinking and speech is not stable and static. There is no rigid correspondence between thought and speech; rather, it is a continuous dynamic interplay. Speech does not express a thought which is ready; it is the thinking that, transforming itself into speech, reorganises and modifies itself, materialising in words.

This discontinuous interrelationship also impacts individual words:

> The discovery of the changeable nature of word meanings and their development is the key to liberating the theory of thinking and speech from the dead end where it currently finds itself. Word meaning is inconstant. It changes during the child's development and with different modes of the functioning of thought. It

> is not a static but a dynamic formation. To establish the changeable nature of meaning, we must begin by defining it correctly. The nature of meaning is revealed in generalization. The basic and central feature of every word is generalization. All words generalize. It is important to emphasize, however, that the fact that the internal nature of word meaning changes implies that the relationship of thought to word changes ... This central idea ... can be expressed in the following general formula: The relationship of thought to the word is not a thing but a process, a movement from thought to word and from word to thought.
>
> *(Vygotsky, 1934; Engl. transl., pp. 249, 250)*

This idea of *processualism*, according to Yarosevsky, is related to Vygotsky's experiences in the theatrical field:

> The notion of a word's significance was not seen as related to its context (as is often supposed), which gives many different shadings or nuances to the word, but to the word's hidden meaning, given to that word by the speaker via his affect and will. Vygotsky derived his notion of hidden meaning from the influence of K. S. Stanislavsky. And again (as with the hypothesis about seeing psychology in the terms of a drama) the art of the theater made a valuable contribution to the science of psychology.
>
> *(Yarosevsky, 1996, p. 172)*

It is important here to note that the contrary also occurred: we can see how psychology has given great support to research on the theatre, the actor, and the public, also with the support drawn from Vygotsky's work. In his works devoted to the topic, especially on the actor (Vygotsky, 1932a), we find numerous ideas of excellent value in theatre criticism.

For example, the ideas on the "sublime moment of the spectator" (Vygotsky, 1925, Chapter 9) or the spectator's triumph, which gave a significant contribution to modern theories of reception. According to it, the audience is not passive but is an active subject whose emotional autonomy needs to be encouraged. As Trimarchi wrote:

> In tragedies we can see some static elements, for example in the hero who has the strength to break a rule considered unavoidable and is then overwhelmed by it. Even in this situation, the situation is dynamic if we think that the hero's fall is accompanied by the "spectator's triumph." Spectators must find a synthesis out of the situation, operated not on a purely cognitive level, but according to a line of "emotional thought." Clearly, the spectator's passivity may be related to other genres, but it does not exist in drama, in the Vygotskyan sense, where the audience is fostered to be frantically active, in search of a synthesis, which is not given *a priori*, among contrasting elements.
>
> *(Trimarchi, 2007, p. 38)*

The ideas of processualism, dialectic action, and "living drama" concern all of Vygotsky's speculations, in particular, the aspects related to inner speech. With concern to the latter, we should consider that once established, inner speech becomes a fundamental element of the human mind. In short, a second level is accomplished, which is inner to speech and lies inside words. According to Vygotsky, *external language is for others, while inner speech is for us, but the difference does not lie in speaking or in the absence of sounds*.

As a fundamental characteristic of inner speech, besides its specific syntax, apparent fragmentation, discontinuity, and abbreviations, there is predicativity. For Vygotsky, predicativity is the fundamental syntactic form of inner speech. In predicativity, the sentence is abbreviated, not because it shortens the number of words using a telegraphic style, but because it tends to preserve the predicate of the sentence and the parts connected to it, omitting the subject and the words linked to it. Verb, in grammar, is the fundamental element of a sentence; it defines an activity, a condition or a quality of the subject. To simplify the concept of predicativity, let us think about what happens among speakers who know a topic and use little words, as they do not have to explain or clarify. Motivations, or rather will, and mostly emotions, are implicit and fundamental.

In the last period of his activity, Vygotsky devoted much energy to the study of emotions, or rather to the emotional and dynamic processes within the interaction between the individual and the environment. This was carried out, as a research program, in the essay *The Problem of Mental Retardation*, published posthumously in 1935, and in the unfinished work *The Theory of Emotions*, begun between 1931 and 1933 and published in 1984. However, paradoxically, his work is best known in the West for his studies on cognitive development. In the last few years, Vygotsky has become one the most studied psychologists of the twentieth century.

He developed an articulated theory of emotions. Vygotsky criticised "the failure of academic psychology that treats only the surface of phenomena" (Vygotsky, 1931–1933, Engl. transl., p. 208).

He was first drawn to psychoanalysis because this Freudian discipline was electively directed to the field of emotions. From a psychoanalytical perspective, this was done by trying to "heroically" preserve the principle of causality in this field. Causal mechanisms, to which Vygotsky refers, are not physicalist decompositions of human biological reality. Emotions and feelings are not elementary, species-specific, genetically fixed functions like in animals. The psychologist refers to complex psychological systems, which have an evolution and cultural-historical connotation, which is connected to the cognitive processes.

In Eisenstein's ideas on inner monologue, we find the ideas of his friend Vygotsky. Inner monologue is modulated by the emotional register. From the encounter of thinking and speech, inner language processes are generated. The inner monologue, outlined by the director, can be considered the analogous formulation, in the field of art, of the process proposed by his Vygotsky. It is part of a drive towards creative activity that is expressed fundamentally in the construction of form.

This always happens based on laws that belong to the dialectic and the development, which is itself dialectical, of the encounter between thinking and speech. A dialectic that, from Engels' perspective, transcends the limits both of individual and social psychology and pre-established knowledge to become a universal method.

In 1925, Vygotsky had already tackled the problem of identifying general criteria to investigate the psychological value of art. It is useful here to go back to the psychologist's ideas and to examine them to understand the conceptual itinerary later followed by Eisenstein. In the words of Vygotsky:

> [...] but it is evident that studying the genesis of art and its dependence on sociological economy is the special subject of the history of art. Art per se, as a well-established trend, as the sum of available works, is an ideology like any other (my italics). Thus, to be or not to be is a problem of method for objective psychology. ... Furthermore, Engels has shown that any ideology is always created with a false consciousness or, essentially, unconsciously. ... Equally futile is the analysis of the emotions of the viewer, since he, too, is shrouded in the psyche's unconsciousness.... One of the first, and easiest, objections against it is the one commonly raised against studying the unconscious by means of psychology. The unconscious, it is said, is by definition something we do not recognize; it is something unknown to us, and therefore it cannot become the subject of scientific investigation. ... This is obviously a superficial approach, since we do study many things of which we have knowledge only from analogies, hypotheses, surmises, etc. ... Accordingly, the work of art, rather than its creator or its audience, should be taken as the basis for analysis. While it is true that a work of art as such is not an object of psychology (having no psyche of its own), we must remember that a historian, studying for instance the French revolution from materials that do not contain any of the objects of his study, finds himself faced with the necessity of actually creating the object of his study by means of indirect, that is, analytic methods. ... [T]he psychologist is forced to resort to material evidence – the works of art – and create a corresponding psychology in order to be able to study the laws governing it. For the psychologist any work of art is a system of stimuli, consciously and intentionally organized in such a way as to excite an aesthetic reaction. ... This method guarantees a sufficient objectivity of results and of investigation, since it proceeds every time from the study of solid, objectively existing, accountable facts. Here is the formula of this method: from the form of the work of art, via the functional analysis of its elements and structure, recreate the aesthetic reaction and establish its general laws.
>
> *(Vygotsky, 1925, pp. 45–48)*

The ideas exposed are mainly related to the characteristics of artistic creation and to the relationship between the work of art and the emotions of the observer. In a broad sense, Vygotsky tries to avoid the complex affective phenomena linked precisely to the creation and enjoyment of art, which is explained with the tools of medical and physiological psychology, Pavlovian or others. This is why, on several occasions, he repeatedly refers to the unconscious, the new concept brought to the attention of the scientific community by psychoanalytical doctrine. The unconscious was the privileged and specific place of passion. The psychologist emphasised how, between the emotions of an animal and those of a civilised man, there is a "leap" that cannot be explained in physiological terms. Vygotsky's thought always revolves around the phenomenon of human history and culture.

The work of art is a device loaded with stimuli that are culturally significant and aimed to evoke typically human emotions, which cannot be explained in an exclusively physiological way;

> Even from the point of view of the most complex affect of a human-like simian closest to man, it is impossible to explain the most elementary human passions. Therefore, causal psychology must break sharply with natural science, causal psychology and seek its own path somewhere outside it and apart from it. As S. Freud says, a completely different approach to the problem of feelings is needed than that which was formed official school of psychology, particularly in medical psychology.
>
> *(Vygotsky, 1931; Engl. transl., p. 208)*

Emotions must be interpreted in cultural-historical terms. If one tries to explain them with an exclusively physiological theory,

> the serious differences that human emotions display depending on the era, the degree of civilization… remain unexplained from the point of view of this theory … Actually, it is impossible to admit that simple perception of a female silhouette automatically evoked an endless series of organic reactions of which could be borne love such as the love of Dante for Beatrice if we do not previously assume the whole ensemble of the theological, political, esthetic, and scientific ideas that comprised the consciousness of the genius, Alighieri.
>
> *(Vygotsky, 1931–1933; Engl. transl., p. 207)*

From these words, it is not difficult to understand that for his theoretical and artistic work, Eisenstein was extremely attracted to Vygotsky's research. There is the idea that a work of art can be composed as a "system of stimuli" that Eisenstein called "attractions" in his early formulations, capable of provoking an aesthetic response in the viewer. Later, in the development of his thought, Eisenstein claims that a work of art can be better understood and described as a dialectical model, according to the mentioned unity of opposites, dynamically overcoming the two opposing poles, the functions of consciousness and the unconscious.

Not forgetting the context, we should remember that Hugo Münsterberg, who studied at the school of Wilhelm Wundt – the founder of experimental psychology – was very interested in film. Münstenberg (1916), who had also worked with William James in film techniques, saw the mechanisms of the higher psychological functions, such as attention, consciousness, will and so on, according to an approach that today we would consider cognitivist. Psychoanalysts considered cinema as an art form capable of triggering the driving forces of the unconscious and making it emerge. Eisenstein tried to combine the two perspectives. The inner monologue can express both the conscious and unconscious dimensions in film montage sequences. Montage is a conscious activity, but, at the same time, in the images, sounds and the linking of the sequences, we also see an organised manifestation which seeks artistic realisation, and it is rooted in the unconscious. Montage presents itself as a linguistic expression that involves the unconscious, according to the laws of inner discourse.

Eisenstein tried to outline dialectically "the general laws" of psyche and art. For this reason, it is necessary to assess the connections between psychoanalytical processes and the structure of montage.

Already in *The Expressive Movement* (1923), Eisenstein saw art as a dialectical expression, simultaneously inner and external, of mind and nature.

At the same time, art is, in a Vygotskyan perspective, an *instrument* which communicates ideological content. Art encounters the human psyche in an analogous way as speech – external to the individual – meets thinking. Therefore, the study of speech, in the Vygotskyan perspective, offers many possibilities for understanding Eisenstein, and he does use these opportunities.

In his analysis, Vygotsky highlights the difference between inner speech, spoken language and written language. Predicativity marks the major difference with written speech, which is the most extensively developed, precise and accurate form of speech when it comes to explication and specification. In a different way, inner speech is the most contracted form of speech, according to Vygotsky.

In this classification, oral language is the intermediate form and may show a tendency towards predicativity when the speakers are familiar with the topic. The concept of predicativity is essential, and it is connected – this must be stressed – to the motivational and emotional dimension of inner speech.

Predicativity has important conceptual implications for Eisenstein's notion of inner monologue. The director is significantly influenced by Vygotsky's "psychology of emotions" (see Didi-Huberman, 2016, p. 311), and it is important to emphasise that predicativity is linked to the emotional dimension. Predicativity rarely belongs to spoken speech, never to written speech and always to inner speech. In other words, the rule of written speech is to be composed of subjects and predicates, whereas in inner speech, the subject is deleted, and the composition is made of predicates.

This "condensation" promotes the dominance of the inner speech, of the "sense" of the word, over its "meaning". Sense is related to the dynamic, emotional, fluctuating, and complex aspects of the word, while "meaning is only one of these zones of the sense that the word acquires in the context of speech. It is the most stable, unified, and precise of these zones" (Vygotsky, 1934; Engl. transl., p. 276). This shifting vagueness of inner speech would be enough, alone, to distinguish it from external speech. In fact, external speech, in both its manifestations, written and oral, remains rigidly connected to the fixity of logical thinking. These distinct aspects, for Vygotsky, make inner speech a "special function" of speech, independent and original.

Vygotsky also describes a phenomenon called *agglutination*, which is conceptually important when examining Eisenstein's ideas. It is a "means of forming unified complex words that are used to express complex concepts" (Vygotsky, 1934; Engl. transl., p. 277). It is because of this characteristic that the sense of words extends dynamically and broadly beyond their simple meaning. The senses of words influence each other, flood into each other. A single word, in the inner speech, can absorb the meaning of previous and subsequent words.

This can also explain a sort of incomprehensibility of inner speech, as differently from the external one, this form of language is not aimed at communication. This "condensation" of inner speech makes it a specific function of the mind, even though it is not alterative to external speech. Inner speech tends to coincide with thinking, but it is a thought where the word, in its semantic value, has "disappeared", or rather it does not correspond to its verbal value. Inner speech is not only made of single words, like external language. It tends to "evaporate" in thought, "Thought is always something whole, something with significantly greater extent and volume than the individual word" (Vygotsky, 1934; Engl. transl., p. 281).

In the words of the psychologist,

> conscience does not evaporate and does not dissolve in pure spirit. Inner speech is speech. It is thought that is connected with the word. However, where external speech involves the embodiment of thought in the word, in inner speech the word dies away and gives birth to thought … Inner speech is a dynamic, unstable, fluid phenomenon that appears momentarily between the more clearly formed and stable poles of verbal thinking, that is, between word and thought.
>
> *(Vygotsky, 1934; Engl. transl., p. 280)*

This conceptual framework echoes Eisenstein's theme of image and movement, which the image holds. Eisenstein perceives the characteristic of inner speech as emerging peculiarities in montage and outlines an analogy between inner speech and inner monologue. Inner monologue is the psychological instrument of montage. It seems that in the inner monologue, the visual part plays a fundamental role, and it is part of the process of communicative elaboration. In this psychological operation, the phenomenon of agglutination represents a significant example. In fact, for analogy, we see how Eisenstein states that montage puts together single frames which cannot be considered in their singularity and distinctness. Agglutination has similar features. According to it, in line with Vygotsky's ideas, in inner speech, there is an overlapping of the meaning of a word with previous or following words.

The fundamental idea is that the form of montage meets the form of thought without neglecting the motivation drive of emotions.

When he introduces the idea of "vertical montage", the term is not to be intended only as a procedure capable of involving the different real perceptive planes, like image and sound.

Technically, for Eisenstein, cinema can be placed at the top of the modern hierarchy of the arts. The film possesses a mental verticality. Metaphorically, cinema – through montage – can descend downwards, where the archaic zone of emotions and drives is located. But it can also ascend upwards, where the area of conscious and intelligent thought is. The result is always intended to be "sensual thought". Montage has the task of bringing the intellectual and emotional dimensions together; "Like no other work of art, film has in montage the especially important prerequisite for direct contact with sensual thought. This is where the chaining force of the film comes from" (Eisenstein, 2002; Ital. transl., vol. I, p. 193).

Eisenstein's cinematographic position on "inner monologue" connected to the concept of inner speech and film montage, technically and perceptively, follows this line. In fact, there is a lack in this elaboration because the passage from word to image is not fully developed. Nevertheless, Eisenstein uses this idea on several occasions in his theoretical elaborations, starting from the moment he speculates on the value of the so-called "intellectual cinema".

As is well known, the theme of "intellectual cinema" was very present, ideologically, in the Soviet world. In intellectual cinema, there was a proposal capable of giving shape, thanks to montage resources, also to abstract concepts and scientific thought constructions. For a certain period, Eisenstein even had the aspiration to transfer Marx's *Capital* on screen.

In Eisenstein's artistic biography, cinema – or rather an intellectual montage – comes after the eccentric and futuristic poetics of "attractions montage", circulating at the time when he engaged in theatre. The passage to intellectual cinema, at the time, also highlighted some limits relative to the previous theoretical ideas. But within this scenario, the theory of inner monologue is suggested as an evolution of intellectual cinema;

> I cite this example to return once more to the intellectual cinema. The specific quality of intellectual cinema was proclaimed to be the content of the film. The trend of thoughts and the movement of thoughts were represented as the exhaustive basis of everything that transpired in the film, i.e., a substitute for the story. Along this line – exhaustive replacement of content – it does not justify itself. And in sequel perhaps to the realization of this, the intellectual cinema has speedily grown a new conception of a theoretical kind: the intellectual cinema has acquired a little successor in the theory of inner monologue.
>
> *(Eisenstein, 1949, p. 129)*

Here, implicitly, Eisenstein acknowledges the capability of inner monologue to face and solve those problems and those rationalistic and ideological excesses that intellectual cinema had, limiting artistic involvement. In his enterprise, Eisenstein welcomes and uses Vygotsky's ideas, not only by virtue of an affinity for the level of concepts. We should never forget that for both, the agreement is always *methodological*; they seek universal methodological criteria. The formal research and the philosophical dialectics of thinking and inner speech intertwine.

Inner monologue becomes an elective instrument in cinema research and realisation, as it looks appropriate in a philosophical sense. In the words of Eisenstein,

> the theory of the inner monologue warned to some extent the ascetic abstraction of the flow of concepts … and herein lies the principal matter with which I wish to deal. Which is - the syntax of inner speech as opposed to that of uttered speech. Inner speech, the flow and sequence of thinking unformulated into the logical constructions in which uttered, formulated thoughts are expressed, has a special structure of its own. This structure is based on a quite distinct series of laws. What is remarkable therein, and why I am discussing it, is that the laws of construction of inner speech turn out to be precisely those *laws which lie at the foundation of the whole variety of laws governing the construction of form and the composition of art-works*. And there is not one formal method that does not prove the split image of one or another law governing the construction exists, which is not a faithful portrait of a determined law governing the construction of inner speech, as distinct from the logic of uttered speech. It could not be otherwise.
>
> *(Eisenstein, 1949, pp. 129, 130)*

The assonance with Vygotsky's thought in this passage is particularly important. To create a work of art, one should follow the same laws of inner speech, which correspond to the stage of sensorial-figurative thinking. This is a Vygotskyan thought that, for the director, *could explain* the sort of "thinking" a work of art "enacts". Inner speech allows the creation of artistic forms, acting as a mediator for those mental processes based on sensation and image. As Montani aptly put it:

> The relation between thinking and artworks is clarified in a definitive way; form and art composition do not show processes of "general thinking" but processes that take place in a particular region of thinking that is organised in an "inner discourse". Between these two universes, in fact, there is a common structure that, nicely put by Eisenstein, is a specific "syntax" characterised by "quite distinct series of laws". It is more likely that in saying so he was referring to the constructive processes of inner discourse discovered by Vygotsky.
>
> *(Montani, 1981, pp. XXVII–XXVIII)*

From a psychological perspective, it is necessary to consider the relation between these processes and some mental criteria used by children and primitive people, and this allows us to understand Eisenstein's interest towards primitive art forms and the way he expressed it in his drawings.

In 1932, after his Mexican experience, Eisenstein had produced a large graphic collection. This is also due to Anita Brenner's invitation as she wanted to publish an article on his drawing in the magazine *Creative Art*.

The idea of *ecstasy* emerges in these works in terms of a state that implies a regression towards forms of thought which come before the rational-logic stage and to the clear differentiation between subject and object. This, among other things, can justify the deformation of proportions contained in some graphical productions, which is coherent with this archaic thought. In a note on *Psychology of Art* (1925a, Chapter 10, note five) by Vygotsky, Ivanov underlined the inclination of Eisenstein towards expressive forms which are not necessarily realistic, in a context where realism had become an ideological duty.

A cognitive role is attributed to ecstasy, and it is referred to as a condition where knowledge is not only an intellectual comprehension, detached from the dialectic of reality, but an emotional and sensitive experience of the dialectic itself;

> In this respect, drawing becomes of primary importance within research which also comprises cinema creation and theoretical reflection: the importance of a dimension in which that dialectic processing that in films is shown in an objective, public form, in theoretical writings is discussed in abstract terms, and is in this case lived subjectively and made productive beyond any limit or inhibition.
>
> *(Somaini, 2011, p. 156)*

Eisenstein kept drawing all his life, from childhood to his last drawing made the night before he died of a heart attack on the tenth of February 1948. He used to make drawings for each one of his film projects. The drawing was a private and autonomous practice for Eisenstein, and at the beginning, it was not meant for public presentation. This private dimension fostered control and expressive potential. It offered the possibility to experiment with expressive forms, free from any constraint. This happened in the Soviet Union in the 1930s and 1940s, where censorship and prohibitions conditioned any work that had to be shown in public.

The interest in hypnosis is connected to the idea of regression. In *General Theory of Montage*, he connects the hypnotic stage to artistic perception, in which regression takes place;

> Hypnosis consists of the same thing and in particular of the fact that it is possible to temporarily neutralise the "superior strata" of conscience. …the hypnotised person is totally subjected to laws of thought and behaviour that, even if controlled by the mental apparatus, act independently from the higher centres.

Anatomically, the behaviour of the mind is in a condition in which the frontal lobes of the brain are excluded. Ontogenetically, it is behaviour that comes before the development of these lobes, at the beginning of their functioning (infantile thought). Phylogenetically, it is behaviour that precedes the historical elaboration of the formal logic thought that required a quite long and troubled evolution of these organs. Pathologically, it is a permanent regression, prolonged or sporadic, caused by a disease or a trauma during the initial stage of mental development. The distinctive trait of this process, within art, will always be its relativity, or rather its acting simultaneously on *two levels*: the regression to a level in which phenomena inherent to this stage are possible and the preservation of the level inherent to conscience.

(Eisenstein, 1985; Ital. transl., p. 148)

6
CONCLUSIONS

The artistic process, with its regressive characteristics, is always a disinhibitory movement of the psyche compared to pure rationality. According to Eisenstein, the phenomenon of psychological regression is also present in religious and magical thinking and in the alterations produced by drugs. In these situations, there is a greater proximity to inner speech to that psychological phenomenon that allows one to perceive internally and then propose externally, in an accessible way, the highest emotional expression. Even the selection of frames has a counterpart in inner speech. Details and close-ups are reserved for those parts of the real world that are perceived as more important or symbolically loaded with the widest meanings. On a more general level, the psychological meaning of the image is under discussion.

This topic attracted Eisenstein a great deal, although, at that time, that kind of consideration, in a psychological domain, was still at an early stage. There are, of course, various physiological aspects that contribute to the study of image psychology, starting with the perceptive process.

Since in this domain, the emotional and dynamic aspects of the relationship with image are central, it is important to refer, first, to the ideas on cinema coming from that part of psychology that is most concerned with emotion: psychoanalysis.

As already observed, historically, psychoanalytical thought made a great contribution to cinema. In the darkness of cinema theatres, emotions develop specific dynamics. Films evoke strong emotions, but it is the cinematographic situation that makes these imaginary stories so meaningful. Psychologically, the screen, more than the theatre stage, gives the spectator a fictional space that holds the characteristics of reality. Cinema *presents*; theatre *represents* (Angelini, 1992, 2014).

Of course, cinema has a great power, but also a *drama performance* has its own effectiveness because in it an unconscious phenomenon takes place – studied by

DOI: 10.4324/9781003398554-7

psychoanalysis and defined as "projective identification" – that cannot be triggered by the screen. The notion of "projective identification" historically comes from Kurt Lewin (1936), who related it to the "psychological field", and it neatly separates the perceptive peculiarities of theatre and cinema. Furthermore, today it provides elements that would delete Eisenstein's concerns regarding the feared invasion of cinema by the theatre due to the introduction of sound.

In psychoanalysis, projective identification indicates the modality through which the subject, the so-called projector, feeds the fantasy, originally unconscious, to move one part of herself/himself to place it in another person, exerting a powerful control over it. The subject who receives this projection, the receiver, is led to conform to and identify with the specific aspect that the projector tends to deposit. It is important to note that it is a process that clearly goes beyond the intrapsychic level to operate on the interpersonal level. The relationship between actor and audience is only one of the examples in which it is possible to apply this concept for interpretative purposes. This relation implies the existence of an interpersonal, intimate, and close relationship of dependency.

In the primitive model of the relation between mother and child, we refer, for example, to the dynamic that exists between patient and analyst, but this is true for all the subjects of any interpsychic relation, including – with due distinction – the relation between theatre, actor, and audience.

Theatre spectators experience an *interpsychic* dynamic, while cinema spectators experience an *intrapsychic* psychodynamic.

The relationship between actor and spectator is physical and concrete. The actor is connected to the audience; or rather, the actor, in order to exist, needs an audience. By virtue of the action performed, actors "expect" the audience to react in a certain way. Actors use their artistic and human strength to achieve this result. If the audience does not react as expected, the actor, artistically and psychologically, surrenders and "dies", "disappearing" from the scene. As they choose to go to the theatre, spectators are certainly inclined to react, fulfilling the actors' wish. Theatre audiences, from the moment they enter the venue until they take their seat, take part in a ritual ceremony that leads them, progressively, to reach a strong emotional relationship with the actors. It is an audience that "wants" to connect mentally with the actors and who wants to be fascinated.

In the past, anyone who had taken an interest in the matter had emphasised the characteristics of "psychic union" that, in performances, takes place between the two subjects.

Ossicini (1973), starting from the evidence of the communication between the actor and the audience and their relationship, introduced the concept of the "psychic field". Based on the above-mentioned ideas, the elementary component of theatrics must be identified in the interpsychic relationship between actor and spectator.

But cinema, where actors do not physically exist, has its own independent power in evoking emotions because it enacts intrapsychic psychodynamics.

Furthermore, the psychological reasons that attract the spectator to the cinema and the theatre are the same. The spectator is interested in theatre and cinema because both tend to satisfy unconscious drives that are forbidden or subject to a strong subjective defence. These are forces that we cannot or do not want to satisfy in real life, but that we cannot fully give up. Cinema and theatre, within certain limits, allow us to approach, in an acceptable form, those impulses that the conscience considers forbidden. It is not a coincidence that, historically and socially, actors have always been the object of criticism and scrutiny from moralists because they are strongly connected to the world of forbidden impulses.

The emotional power cinema retains, on a psychological level, has often been linked to the power of dreams, but this comparison is far too obvious and limited.

Studies on film perception, developed throughout the twentieth century, were connected to different psychological disciplines. The most famous connection is to the Gestalt school and to psychoanalysis, which evolved progressively in other fields. The perceptual problem of movement, the cinematic representation of time and space, the effects of framing and camera movements, the potential meaning of editing techniques, the psychodynamics of the spectator, the implications in the field of social psychology, etc. are topics that were all studied and investigated.

The physiological psychology of film perception has carried out several analyses, ranging from the study of specialised neurons and the analysis of individual movement characteristics of visual *stimuli* to the spectator's eye-tracking and so on. For researchers, film was a scientific tool to study human beings, as many great psychologists demonstrated. Among the many scholars, we should mention Pavlov, Köhler, Lewin, Spitz, Lorenz, and others who resorted to cinema both to illustrate their discoveries and to identify their research "data". Cinematic perception, in many respects, is a field that still has a long way to go in terms of interesting results.

The cinematic situation, with respect to time and space, places the spectator in an imaginary world, out of reality and human life. Historical developments in the language of film (rhythm, type of shots, editing, colour, sound, electronics, etc.) progressively changed the perceptive abilities of the spectator. The brain of the contemporary spectator is identical, anatomically, to that of the spectator who saw the first Méliès films at the end of the nineteenth century, but the historical and technological context is different, and for this reason, cinema is different.

According to Luria, brain functions aimed at film perception are also *historicised*. Today, viewers possess perceptual abilities, also fed by television and new media networks, that are different from their predecessors and are submitted to frequent and strenuous adaptations. On the contrary, for the newly born, by virtue of the historicisation of brain functions, the perceptive context, cinema, and media in general become an accepted and ordinary *datum*, one of the elements that contribute to the individual's development. This is one of the ways in which cinema, within its limits, modifies human history. Aleksandr Luria, beginning with the studies of Vygotsky, deepened this type of psychophysiological theoretical perspective (Luria, 1962).

From a cinematographic perspective, this psychophysiological dimension modifies the very criteria of *the spectacular*, both with respect to filming and editing techniques and with respect to the narrative criteria with which the story is conceived, dramaturgically, in the film. From a psychological perspective, cinema – throughout its history and its technological and linguistic development – has always had the extraordinary ability to place us emotionally outside the ordinary and the familiar.

It is useful to outline an elementary timeline of this historical medium:

1 *The first Cinema*, with Lumière and Méliès, was a machine of *wonders* that thrilled without real narrative development.
2 *Classic Cinema*, in which we can place Eisenstein's work. From the 1920s to the 1950s, along with the advent of sound, classic cinema explored and developed the power of narration, especially in Hollywood. In this period, cinema freed itself from a social image of a playful kind to qualify itself as true art (Arnheim, 1933–1938).
3 *Modern Cinema* dates from the post-war period to the 1980s. It claims the supremacy of *consciousness* expressed through different modalities. It is the triumph of signature film and a great source for psychoanalysts who delved into the works of Alfred Hitchcock and Orson Wells, and then into Neorealism, the Nouvelle Vague, and all the "New Cinema" of the 1960s and 1970s. The number of authors is endless, but, from the psychoanalytical point of view, we should at least remember Truffaut, Bergman, Antonioni, Fellini, Tarkovsky, Allen, Bertolucci, etc. Modern cinema calls on the spectator to be mentally committed, or assume a critical attitude, towards the film.
4 *Contemporary Cinema*, or the primacy of *sensations*. Originating in the 1980s, it is still a phenomenon. It is the cinema of special effects, of large multiplexes (which was significantly impacted by the COVID-19 pandemic) of technology that does not need a reality to be filmed to produce a completely self-sufficient world of images. It is a cinema strongly influenced in its language and narrative structures by video games. *The spectacular* is paramount; the film aims to strike and impress; it retains a sort of Neo-Baroque style. Obviously, in any spectacular-type proposal, the more obvious the ideas, the more the impact of sensory stimuli must be enhanced.

It is also interesting to consider that the conditions of cinema fruition are changing. With content providers, it is possible to see films, even recent ones, at home. Thus, the ritual part of entering the cinema in that case is not possible, while it still exists for theatregoers.

From a historical perspective, as mentioned, the emotional aspects of cinema have been the chosen ground of psychoanalysis. Cesare Musatti (1963) came to define the phenomenon of "attacks of cinematic anxiety", but these are limited cases connected to the phobia of cinema. There is a psychoanalytical approach aimed at studying the psychodynamics of the spectator at the cinema. From this perspective, it has emerged that, in viewers, the motion picture event achieves its psychological influence through two fundamental mechanisms. On the one hand, *projection*, that is to say, that process according to which we attach to the actors' ideas and aspirations that are ours, even if they are not actualised; on the other hand, *identification*, through which the viewer assimilates aspects and feelings of the actors (see Angelini, 1992, Chapter 5). These two psychodynamic mechanisms should not be confused with *projective identification*, which is a typical phenomenon of *theatre*. Identification can be so intense as to lead cinema spectators, especially in an evolutive age, to imitate their idols in behaviour and clothing. The effects of these psychodynamic mechanisms on the public are, in a classic psychoanalytical perspective, essentially two: *catharsis* and *suggestion*. The term *catharsis* is a Greek word that means "purification". In psychotherapy, the cathartic method aims to achieve the effect of "purification" through an adequate discharge, or abreaction, of the pathogenic effects. *Suggestion* is the process through which a person is influenced to the point of accepting other people's ideas, beliefs, and thoughts. It was observed that suggestive elements are an essential component of the hypnotic phenomenon. The suggestive strength of the film is enhanced by the situation in the venue: in the dark, as in dreams, when physical contact with the environment is limited and the person is in a comfortable situation. The viewers, with their attention fully on the screen, by virtue of the multiple physical and mental processes, are in a situation that was defined as "paranoid relaxation". The comparison with dreams is intended in an analogical sense. Psychoanalysis has always loved art and pondering on meaning of images. From a psychoanalytical perspective, thinking in images differs from realistic or conceptual thinking, being closer to the individual's driving sources. This thought, consequently, is less coherent with the principle of reality aimed at the activity of the conscious self and, paradoxically, more real on an emotional level. Eisenstein supported analogous concepts in his personal elaboration. In the domain of psychodynamic phenomena, the suggestive aspect leads the viewer to accept more easily the violent and erotic elements on the screen. They foster the "cathartic effect", a sort of psychological happiness. Both dream and cinema represent, in fact, forms of evasion from the real world. Both situations, cinema and oneiric allow, at least partially, us to lose control over ourselves. In other words, due to the cathartic effect, the spectator experiments with a psychological fulfilment aimed to establish a balance that the unconscious drives would tend to alter. On the other hand, for its suggestive effect, the viewer is also fostered to more easily accept those erotic and violent elements depicted on the screen; the search could consequently return, in diversely accentuated forms, also in real life. This affective mobilisation evoked by cinema represents, since its birth, a problem that society has tried to face with the aid of censorship. Stalin was fully aware of the suggestive and propagandistic power of cinema. His acts of censorship even occurred first-hand, as was the case with Eisenstein's *General Line*. We see that, in politically authoritarian situations, as in Stalinism and Nazism, with their enormous historical differences, censorship helped to contain any possible dissent. In those situations, cinema was mostly conceived, in an instrumental way, as a means to build consensus. Later, in the democracies of the second half of the last century, the object of censorship was mainly sexuality.

Today, in cinema as well as in the media, a sort of sexual pseudo-liberation gives the illusion that sexual conflicts have been overcome, finally. But the reality in which we live is not what it seems to be; it is not a free and tolerant society that, as such, does not produce that pseudo-hypersexuality with inhibition, which was typical of nineteenth-century hysteria. Instead, we observe an ambivalent society that appears pseudo-hypersexual and is in turn inhibited in its ability to genuinely enjoy sexuality. Although being exhibited and homologated in the media, sexuality continues to carry a load of transgression and scandal, with strong super-egoic reactions. Moreover, the feeling of transgression in art and cinema does not only involve sexuality. Eisenstein's problems with Stalin's regime were not generated by the sexual contents of his films but by the aesthetical and more generally ideological meaning (Angelini, 2020, p. 201). On the other hand, on a psychoanalytical level, even defending ideas and beliefs implies a strong drive load and can be connected to instincts. Through identification and projection, cinema stimulates instincts. Authorities of any kind have always perceived that both cinema and theatre are very close to the world of instincts and drive. With concern to the mentioned effects on the spectator, catharsis and suggestion, we should observe that most parts of the situations that allow catharsis can promote, simultaneously, suggestion. There is no cathartic action without a strong identification, but the identification is also the basis of suggestive action. The value of the two different actions is dialectical, and it is related to the different personalities of the spectators. Films that attract more audience are those in which there are hidden factors that act on the deep strata of our minds. Factors that we cannot or do not want to satisfy in real life but which we cannot give up fully.

Within certain limits, films fulfil in an innocuous way those drives that conscience considers prohibited. This explains why, in cinema, erotism and violence have such a huge space. Even if we are not always ready to acknowledge it, erotic and aggressive themes, in general passions, draw our interest. Referring to some exclusive characteristics of cinema representation, as pointed out by Eisenstein when talking about hypnosis, the spectator at the cinema is in front of a fictional space that has the characteristics of reality but is, objectively, in no place. From a psychoanalytical perspective, Musatti (1969) highlighted the different ways in which a story can be experienced in a novel, at the theatre, or at the cinema. For novel readers, the facts described are imagined. It is an exclusively mental and subjective *representation*. In theatre, the spectator perceives a portion of real space, namely the stage, and through the sets, costumes, gestures, and actors' speeches, a fictional reality is presented, but theatre spectators *pretend* it is real. At the cinema, the spectator experiences a sort of immediate perception that *seems real* and in which facts are directly *presented*.

Historically, different authors have concentrated their attention on the superior realistic power of cinema. C. Metz wrote: "the theatrical fiction is experienced more … whereas cinematic fiction is experienced rather as the quasi-real presence of that unreal itself" (Metz, 1977; Engl. transl., p. 70). The greater influence of cinema on the audience, compared to any other kind of entertainment, is due to the ability of the cinematic situation to carry the spectator into another dimension. This powerful *character of cinematic reality* needs to be analysed when considering this medium's artistic potential. Cinema can keep the spectator's participation even beyond actual artistic values. In contrast, the drop of attention during an uninteresting theatre performance is fast and inevitable. Of course, this aspect does not add to or take away from the capability of artistic expression in cinema. Like any other expressive form, it may or may not reach artistic levels in relation to the skills of the author and the material used.

The analogy between the cinematographic and oneiric situations in which dreams are experienced was highlighted mostly by authors who had an interest in psychoanalysis, like Musatti (1963, 1969). Eisenstein recognised the capability of cinema to provoke a psychological regression in the spectator, but dream and film situations cannot be juxtaposed.

There are obvious differences, along with analogies. First, both cinema and dreams lead the individual to experiment with a different situation from real life. In both situations, this is possible only if the individual suspends, temporarily, the course of his normal life. Dreaming occurs while sleeping when physical contact with the environment is limited. We have already mentioned that the detachment from the outside world of people who go to sleep has some analogies with the darkness in cinemas and with the comfortable seats. The fundamental aspect is, simplifying, that both dream and cinema represent forms of evasion from the real world. Compared to the dream, there are still, of course, differences in the situation experienced by the spectator, who is passive towards images. Nevertheless, the juxtaposition between dream and reality shows analogies with that between cinema and reality. Dreams, like films, are easily forgotten and modified in the act of remembering them. They both lack the solid references provided by real life. Additionally, time and space in cinema are, as mentioned, different from real life. According to Eisenstein, time and space must be organised according to the inner monologue that, in montage, creates the film. According to Freud, the time and space of the dream are dominated by instinctual forces that, due to censorship, make images emerge only in exchange for a severe symbolic toll.

In film, the task of the director is to conceive and create a sequence of shots where the images transfer the message envisioned by the director in a rationally coherent and emotionally poignant way. The emotional aspect is fundamental. The *vexata quaestio*, according to which cinema is compared to dreams, is reduced to the fact that the drive matter that feeds dreams and cinema is the same: desire.

The emotional drive, the emotional matter that motivates the functioning of inner monologue, was a constant interest of Eisenstein when studying the psychological aspects of cinema. The director developed this theme with the theoretical tools of his era.

> Only the film-element commands a means for an adequate presentation of the whole course of thoughts through a disturbed mind. Or, if literature can do it, it is only a literature that breaks through the limits of its orthodox enclosure. Literature's most brilliant achievement on this field has been the immortal "inner monologues" of Leopold Bloom in *Ulysses*. When Joyce and I met in Paris, he was intensely interested in my plans for the inner-film-monologue, with a far broader scope than is afforded by literature … The "inner monologue", as a literary method of abolishing the distinction between subject and object in stating the hero's reexperience in a crystallized form, is first observed by research-workers in literary experiment as early as 1887… It finds full expression, however, only in the cinema. For only the sound-film is capable of reconstructing all phases and all specifics of the course of thoughts … As if presenting inside the characters the inner play, the conflict of doubts, the explosion of passion, the voice of the reason reasoning… How fascinating it is to listen to one's own train of thought … the syntax of inner speech as distinct from outer speech. The quivering inner words that correspond with the visual images … To listen and to study, in order to understand structural laws and assemble them into an inner monologue construction ... How obvious it becomes that material of the sound-film is not dialogue. *The true material of the sound-film is, of course, the monologue* … the montage form, as a structure, is a reconstruction of the laws of the thought process.
>
> *(Eisenstein, 1949, p. 106)*

The implicit idea is that, in the structure of a work of art, events do not follow a straight line. Ivanov, in a note on *Psychology of Art* (Vygotsky, 1915, Chapter 7, p. 324, note five), stated that this conviction of Eisenstein's was close to Vygotsky's ideas.

In *Nonindifferent Nature*, Eisenstein wrote: "Classic examples of a similar nonsequential narration could be, for Russian literature, the *Pistol Shot* by Pushkin, which starts narration from the middle, *Light Breathing by* Iv. Bunin, and a huge quantity of other models" (1981; Ital. transl., p. 312). These were the same authors cited by Vygotsky on the same topic. According to Ivanov, this showed that Eisenstein knew the manuscript of his psychologist friend on art psychology. The stream of thinking, which is not mechanically linear, rules over montage form, but this process is governed by precise laws: "Logic obeys a whole series of laws in its constructions, so, equally, this inner speech, this sensual thinking, is subject to no clear-cut laws and structural peculiarities" (Eisenstein, 1949, p. 130).

These precise laws, which are dialectical laws,

> are known, and in the light of the considerations here set out, represent an inexhaustible storehouse, as it were, of laws for the construction of form, the study

> and analysis of which have immense importance in the mastering the "mysteries" of technique of form. For the first time we are placed in possession of a firm storehouse of postulates, bearing on *what* happens to the initial thesis of the theme when it is translated into a chain of sensorial images.
>
> *(Eisenstein, 1949, p. 130)*

Dialectically, we simultaneously reach reason and sentiments, the superior and profound strata of psyche. The means is a work of art capable of generating, simultaneously, the impact of form and content. In art, like in psychology, the relation between subject and object had, for Eisenstein, a dynamic character, clearly dialectical. This is the "evolutive pattern" both in the domain of conscience and the creation of artworks. In psychology, the path that leads from the elementary functions to the higher psychological functions is dialectical. These are the functions of thought, but their motivation belongs to the sphere of feelings. In art, the pattern that, by adding qualitatively different expressive elements, leads to the creation of an organic artwork, i.e., the artistic synthesis, is dialectical. As mentioned, with the term organic, we point to the continuity between the inorganic matter of artwork and the different forms of life. Artworks under the same laws that regulate the evolution of art and history. In this perspective, following Vygotsky and again dialectically, in art as in psychological functioning, the "inactive and rudimental" functions of consciousness survive as "remnants" of the historical development of behaviour. In this way, there is a line that holds together the past and the present, the higher and primitive stages of consciousness. According to Eisenstein, art manifests fundamentally in this possibility. Even from this idea of simultaneity emerges the idea of a "spheric book", which can be read starting from each single part but can include any other artistic expression. The double temporal dimension is in line with the dialectic and with Vygotsky's notion of consciousness, which considers art as a historical product of human expressive ability. This is connected to a model of individual history, made of conflicts and qualitative leaps, that, with new acquisitions, never loses track of past events. Likewise, a thought capable of generalisation must not lose the various parts, even if they do not identify with the whole, continuing to be part of a more complex dialectical synthesis. Art is the expressive form of a movement that belongs both to the interior reality of consciousness and to the external reality of nature and history.

As Eisenstein wrote:

> The dialectic of works of art is built upon a most curious "dual-unity." The effectiveness of a work of art is built upon the fact that there takes place in it a dual process: an impetuous progressive rise along the lines of the highest explicit steps of consciousness and a simultaneous penetration by means of the structure of the form into the layers of profoundest sensual thinking. The polar separation of these two lines of flows creates that remarkable tension of unity of form and content characteristic of true art-works. Apart from this there are no true art-works.
>
> *(Eisenstein, 1949, pp. 144, 145)*

This unity between feeling and expressive moment, already found in Vygotsky, shifts the engine, and equally the compass, of communicative linguistic effort towards the basic area of emotions. According to Vygotsky, several concepts exist at once as multiple elements of a "cloud". They only unfold in the external language at a later stage. Therefore, what motivates thought cannot be 'another thought' and certainly cannot be language in its verbal form. Motivational elements of thinking, according to Vygotsky, are those that mostly evoke Eisenstein's interest, the emotional aspects. Intrinsic factors that give motivation and meaning to the process of inner speech are emotions. They push this process towards mediation and verbal expression. What motivates thought does not come from concepts or grammar but from an area of the human psyche that the director advocates and artistically searches for emotions and desires. In Vygotsky's psychology, there is the idea that, at the basis of each thought, there is an emotional and determined motivation (see Vygotsky, 1931–1933); in thinking there, is an innate "physiological" element, in an emotional sense. Vygotsky suggests that inner speech, the closest to the form of thought not yet verbalised, is the most emotionally charged; thought

> is not borne of other thoughts. Thought has its origin in the motivating sphere of consciousness, a sphere that includes our inclinations and needs, our interests and impulses, and our affect and emotion. The affective and volitional tendency stands behind thought. Only here do we find the answer to the final "why" in the analysis of thinking. A true and complex understanding of another's thought becomes possible only when we discover its real, affective-volitional basis.
>
> *(Vygotsky, 1934; Engl. Transl., p. 282)*

In the essay *Educational Psychology* (1926), the psychologist has put forward the problem of "education of emotional behaviour". Vygotsky stated that, psychologically, a sort of desire must precede any new knowledge, something that resembles "the philosopher's wonder" the Greeks talked about. Every educational endeavour works if it has, as a starting point, a certain degree of emotional involvement and a dimension that is sensitive to affectivity. Vygotsky acknowledges the importance of emotions in guiding and informing cognition (see 1926, Chapter 6).

Inner monologue generates from a constantly evolving process that has, at its basis, an emotional motivation. The affective drive promotes the generation of a strongly emotional, though not yet verbalised. It is a process that, from the affective motivation at the origin of thought, through inner speech, moves outward, creating the external formulation of thought in words. A progressive pattern that, from "inside", leads to "outside" and dialectically keeps open the regressive movement towards the inside;

> In our analysis, verbal thinking has emerged as a complex dynamic whole where the relationship *between* thought and word is manifested as a movement through several internal plans, as a transition from one plane to another. We have carried our analysis from the most external to the most internal plane. In the living drama of verbal thinking, movement takes the reverse path. It moves from

> the motive that gives birth to thought, to the formation of thought itself, to its mediation in the internal word, and finally, to words themselves. However. It would be a mistake to imagine that this simple path from thought to word is always realized. On the contrary, the current state of knowledge indicates that extremely varied direct and reverse movements and transitions from one plane to another are possible ... However, our task was not to study the varied movements that are realized along the trajectory from thought to word. Our goal was merely to show that the relationship between thought and word is a dynamic process. It is a path from thought to word, a completion and embodiment of the thought in the word.
>
> *(Vygotsky, 1934; Engl. transl., p. 283)*

In this complex pattern, in which there are different and simultaneous psychological re-organisations of the mind, affections are at the basis. However, affections are included in the historical and cultural dimension and, in their development, re-organise themselves; "The historical development of affects or emotions resides mainly in the fact that the original connections become changed and that a new order and new connections develop" (Vygotsky, 1930b; Engl. transl., p. 126).

Emotions must be considered as an example of systemic organisation and cannot be studied independently from cognitive processes. According to Vygotsky, emotions exist only from a reductionist and naturalistic perspective, but in this case, their connection to higher psychological functions is not acknowledged, particularly memory, thinking, and speech.

In light of what was mentioned, inner speech is maintained in the form of a thought not yet verbalised and strongly connotated on an emotional level. It is a passage in which visual imagination can play a significant role. In supporting this perspective, Eisenstein, almost analogously paraphrasing Vygotsky, elaborates on the idea of "inner monologue".

The mental realisation of a film, the editing the director conducts in imagination, uses the inner monologue that takes place in the specificity of the Vygotskyan inner speech. This primitive inner speech is emotionally loaded, redundant of specific affective elements, and full of visual suggestions. It is for this reason that Eisenstein considered cinema as the most effective and powerful artistic means for the inner development of "sensual thinking". Mind is motivated by emotions and works according to them. Images transfer contents in a direct way. As Eisenstein states, cinema is "a genuinely synthetic art – an art of organic synthesis in its very essence, not a 'concert' of co-existent, contiguous, 'linked', but actually independent arts ... the method of cinema, when fully comprehended, will enable us to reveal an understanding of the method of art in general" (Eisenstein, 1949, pp. 193, 194). He believes that the inner laws of cinema composition can be the same that regulate communicative and expressive capabilities.

In cinema, as in any other art, in a dialectical way, form must emotionally express conceptual content, but for Eisenstein, conceptual content is *ideological*. A contemporary figure to the director, Boris Fridman, a member of the Russian Psychoanalytic Society, obtained meaningful results studying ideologies from a psychoanalytical perspective. The theoretical assumptions of this author, coming from Marxism, echoed the ideas of Vygotsky and Eisenstein. Ideology exists mainly in the cultural and historical dimensions. It keeps together, simultaneously, the individual's social and emotional contents (see Fridman, 1925).

This need also belongs to cinema, which, as an excellence among arts, has the task of putting in communication, dialectically, similar forces.

Artwork, like inner speech, must connect emotion and will, or motivational forces, with the manifested expression it proposes in the external world. Cinema, according to Eisenstein, is not only "the most advanced of arts", but it is also the best tool to detect more directed methodological criteria to give life to an art that is valuable and real. In the words of Eisenstein, "we have to tend towards an expressive and effective form, to the highest degree, and use the simplest and most economical form to express what we want" (Eisenstein, 2002; Ital. transl., p. 109).

In Eisenstein's perspective, artwork – both in its expression and in its study – was set within an extraordinarily strong ethical tension. Like many artists, scientists, and psychologists, contemporary to him, he generously believed himself able to change the world with his work tools. The commitment to artistic production was, first of all, a means to create the Soviet "New Man" and transform society from its foundations. The horizon of this project had the same limits as the October Revolution. Eisenstein hoped for a future that was possible, even if not yet feasible, capable of producing art and a cinema that embraced the entire human experience and contributed to improving it in a real and ideal sense.

BIBLIOGRAPHY[1]

Note for the readers: the original names' transliteration used in the specific reference has been added in square brackets.

Adler, M. (1904). *Kausalität und Teleologie im Streite um die Wissenschaft*. Wien: Brand.
Adler, M. (1930–1931). *Lehrbuch der materialistischen Geschichtsauffassung*, vol. 2. Wien: Laub.
Alexander, F. (1923). 'Der biologische Sinn psychologischer Vorgänge (Über Buddhas Versenkungslehre)'. *Imago*, 9 (1), pp. 35–57.
Aleksandrov, G. V., Eisenstein, S. M. and Pudovkin, V. I. (1928). 'A Statement on the Sound-Film', in Eisenstein, S. M. (1949). *Film Form: Essays in Film Form* (edited and translated by J. Leyda). Pp. 257–261. New York: Harcourt, Brace, & World.
Angelini, A. (1983). *Influenza della rivoluzione industriale sulle origini del cinema*. Roma: Ed. Associazione Italiana di Cinematografia Scientifica.
Angelini, A. (1988). *La psicoanalisi in Russia*. Napoli: Liguori.
Angelini, A. (1989). 'Psicologia della percezione e del montaggio cinematografico in Rudolf Arnheim and Sergej M. Ejzenštejn: Due ipotesi a confronto'. *Storia della psicologia e delle scienze del comportamento*, 1 (giugno), pp. 49–60.
Angelini, A. (1992). *Psicologia del cinema*. Napoli: Liguori.
Angelini, A. (1996). *Otto Fenichel: psicoanalisi, politica e società*. Bologna: Cosmopoli.
Angelini, A. (2002). *Pionieri dell'inconscio in Russia*. Napoli: Liguori.
Angelini, A. (2008). 'History of the Unconscious in Soviet Russia: From its Origins to the Fall of the Soviet Union'. *International Journal of Psychoanalysis*, 89, pp. 369–388.
Angelini, A. (2009). *Un enciclopedista romantico*. Napoli: Liguori.
Angelini, A. (2013). 'On the Ten Letters by Sigmund Freud to Wilhelm Reich (1924–1930)'. *The Italian Psychoanalytic Annual*, VIII, 2014.
Angelini, A. (2014). *Psicoanalisi e arte teatrale*. Roma: Alpes Ed.
Angelini, A. (2019). *Otto Fenichel: Psicoanalisi, metodo e storia*. Roma: Alpes Ed.
Angelini, A. (2020). 'Sergej M. Ejzenštejn, la psicologia e la psicoanalisi'. *Psicoterapia e Scienze Umane*, 54 (2), pp. 199–234.

Aumont, J. (1979). *Montage Eisenstein*. Paris: Albatros.
Arnheim, R. (1933–1938). *Film as Art*. Berkeley and Los Angeles: University of California Press, 1964.
Avenarius, R. (1888/1890). *Kritik der reinen Ehrfahrung*, vol. 2. Leipzig: Fuels.
Bakhurst, D. (2007). '*Vygotsky's Demons*,' in Daniels, H., Cole, M. and Wertsch, J. (eds.). *The Cambridge Companion to Vygotskij*. Pp. 50–77. New York: Cambridge University Press.
Baldwin, J. M. (1913). *History of Psychology: A Sketch and an Interpretation*. London: Watts.
Benjamin, W. (1928). *One-Way Street*, in Michael, W. Jennings (ed.). Cambridge, MA: Belknap Press of Harvard University Press. 2016.
Bertetto, P. (ed.) (1975). *Ejzenštejn FEKS Vertov: Teoria del cinema rivoluzionario*. Milano: Feltrinelli.
Blonsky, P. P. (1925). 'Psichologya kak nauka o povedenii', in *Izbrannye psikhologicheskie proizvedeniya* (*Selected Psychological Writings*). Moscow: Akad. Pedag. Nauk RSFSR, 1964.
Bordwell, D. (1993). *The Cinema of Eisenstein*. Cambridge, MA: Harvard University Press.
Bulgakova, O. (1989). *Herausforderung Ejzenštejn*. Berlin and Cambridge, MA: Akademie der Künste.
Bulgakova, O. (1998). *Eisenstein und Deutschland. Texte. Dokumente, Briefe*. Berlin: Henschel Verlag.
Bulgakowa, O. (2001). 'La conférence berlinoise d'Eisenstein: entre la psychanalyse et la gestalt- psychologie', in Chateau, D., Jost, F. and Lefebvre. M. (eds.). *Eisenstein: L'ancien et le nouveau*. Pp. 171–183. Paris: Publications de la Sorbonne.
Caroli, D. and Mecacci, L. (2020). 'Forbidden Science: The Dismantling of Pedology and the Listing of the Works of Pedologists in the Soviet Union in 1936–1938'. *European Yearbook of the History of Psychology*, 6, pp. 11–61.
Carroll, J. M. (1980). *Toward a Structural Psychology of Cinema*. The Hague, Paris and New York: Mouton Publishers.
Cassirer, E. (1923–1929). *The Philosophy of Symbolic Forms*, vol. 4. New Haven, CT and London: Yale University Press, 1953–1996.
Cervini, A. (2006). *Sergej M. Ejzenštejn: L'immagine estatica*. Roma: Ente dello Spettacolo.
Cervini, A. (2010). *La ricerca del metodo*. Milano-Udine: Mimesis.
Chateau, D., Jost, F. and Lefebvre, M. (eds.) (2001). *Ejzenštejn: l'ancien et le nouveau*. Paris: Publications de la Sorbonne.
Cole, M. (1979). 'A Portrait of Luria,' in Luria, A. R. (ed.). *The Making of Mind: A Personal Account of Soviet Psychology*. Cambridge, MA: Harvard University Press.
Conquest, R. (1973). *The Great Terror: Stalin's Purges of the Thirties*. Revised edition. New York: Collier Books.
D'Arco, S. A. (ed.) (1980). *La cultura nella tradizione russa del XIX e XX secolo*. Torino: Einaudi.
De Benedictis, M. (2001). *Ejzenštejn. Fino all'ultima estasi*. Roma: Lithos
Deborin, A. M. (1924). *'G. Lukács and his Criticism of Marxism'*, in 'Word Socialist Web Site'.
Deborin, A. M. (1928). 'Ein neuer Feldzug des Marxismus'. *Unter dem Banner des Marxismus*, 2 (1–2), pp. 44–67.
Deleuze, G. (1983). *Cinema 1: The Movement Image*. London and New York: The Athlone Press.

Del Rio, P. and Alvarez, A. (2007). 'Inside and Outside the *Zone of Proximal Development*: An Ecofunctional reading of Vygotsky', in Daniels, H., Cole, M. and Wertsch, J. (eds.). *The Cambridge Companion to Vygotskij*. Pp. 276–303. New York: Cambridge University Press.

De Saussure, F. (1922). *Course in General Linguistics*. La Salle, Illinois: Open Court.

Didi-Huberman, G. (2016). 'Pathos and Praxis (Eisenstein versus Barthes),' in Kleiman, N. and Somaini, A. (eds.). *Sergei M. Eisenstein: Notes for a General History of Cinema*. Amsterdam: Amsterdam University Press.

Eisenstein [Ejzenštejn], S. M. (1932–1933). '*La regia: l'arte della messa in scena*,(Montani, P. ed.). Venezia: Marsilio, 1989.

Eisenstein, S. M. (1934). 'Through Theater to Cinema', in Eisenstein, S. M. *Film Form: Essays in Film Form* (edited and translated by J. Leyda). Pp. 3–17. New York: Harcourt, Brace, & World.

Eisenstein, S. M. (1935). 'Film Forms: New Problems', in Eisenstein, S. M. *Film Form: Essays in Film Form* (edited and translated by J. Leyda). Pp. 122–149. New York: Harcourt, Brace, & World.

Eisenstein [Ejzenštejn], S. M. (1938). 'Montaggio 1938', in Ejzenštejn, S. M. *Il montaggio* (Montani P. ed.). Pp. 89–127. Venezia: Marsilio, 1986.

Eisenstein [Ejzenštejn], S. M. (1940a). 'Il montaggio verticale', in Ejzenštejn, S. M. *Il montaggio* (Montani P. ed.). Pp. 129–214. Venezia: Marsilio, 1986.

Eisenstein, S. M. (1940b). 'The Psychology of Art', in Eisenstein, S. M. *The Psychology of Composition* (Upchurch, Alaned ed.). Pp. 1–15. Methuen, Calcutta and London: Seagull Books, 1988.

Eisenstein, S. M. (1946). 'Pré-natal experience', in Ejzenštejn, S. M. *Memorie: La mia arte nella vita* (Montani, P. ed.). Pp. 358–359. Venezia: Marsilio, 2006.

Eisenstein, S. M. (1949). *Film Form: Essays in Film Form* (edited and translated by J. Leyda). New York: Harcourt, Brace & World.

Eisenstein, S. M. (1963–1970). *Izbrannye proizvedeniya v shesti tomakh* (Selected Works in six volumes), in Kleiman, N. (ed.). Moscow: Iskusstvo.

Eisenstein, S. M. (1964). *Forma e tecnica del film e lezioni di regia*, in Gobetti, P. (ed.), reprinted 2003. Torino: Einaudi.

Eisenstein [Ejzenštejn], S. M. (1981). *La natura non indifferente*, in Montani, P. (ed.). Venezia: Marsilio.

Eisenstein [Ejzenštejn], S. M. (1985). *Teoria generale del montaggio*, in Montani, P. (ed.). Venezia: Marsilio.

Eisenstein [Ejzenštejn], S. M. (1986a). *Il montaggio*, in Montani, P. (ed.). Venezia: Marsilio.

Eisenstein, S. M. (1986b). *Eisenstein on Disney*, in Leyda, J. (ed.). London: Methuen.

Eisenstein, S. M. (1988). *The Psychology of Composition*, in Upchurch, A. (ed.). London: Methuen.

Eisenstein, S. M. (1995). *Beyond the Stars: The Memoirs of Sergei Eisenstein*. London: British Film Institute.

Eisenstein, [Ejzenštejn] S. M. (1997). *Memorie*. Venezia: Marsilio, 2006.

Eisenstein, [Ejzenštejn] S. M. (1998). *Il movimento espressivo*. Venezia: Marsilio, 1989.

Eisenstein, S. M. (2002). *Metod*, in Kleiman N. (ed.), vol. 2. Moscow: Muzej Kino.

Eisenstein [Ejzenštejn], S. M. (2009). *Sulla biomeccanica. Azione scenica e movimento*, in Cervini, A. (ed.). Roma: Armando.

Eisenstein [Ejzenštejn], S. M. (2020). *II Metodo*: vol. I (A. Cervini ed.), ebook. Venezia: Marsilio.

Ellenberger, H. F. (1970). *The Discovery of the Unconscious: The History and Evolution of Dynamic Psychiatry*. New York: Basic Books.
Engels, F. (1878). *Antidühring: Herr Eugen Dühring's Revolution in Science*. Moscow: Progress, 1977.
Engels, F. (1925). *Dialectics of Nature*. New York: International Publishers, 1940.
Eppensteiner, B., Fallend, K. and Reichmayr, J. (1987). 'Die Psychoanalyse im Film 1925/26 (Berlino/Vienna)', *Psiche*, 41 (2), pp. 129–139.
Etkind, A. (1993). *Eros of the Impossible: The History of Psychoanalysis in Russia*. Boulder, CO: Westview Press, 1997.
Fenichel, O. (1934). 'Psychoanalysis as the Nucleus of a Future Dialectical-Materialistic Psychology', *American Imago*, 24, 1967, pp. 290–311.
Ferenczi, S. (1924). *Thalassa: A Theory of Genitality*. Broadway, Albany, New York: *Psychoanalytic Quarterly*, 1938.
Ferruta, A. (ed.) (2005). 'Configurazioni iconiche e pensabilità', in Ferruta, A. (ed.). *Pensare per immagini*. Pp. 25–42. Roma: Borla.
Fracassi, C. (1977). *Aleksandra Kollontaj e la rivoluzione sessuale*. Roma: Editori Riuniti.
Freud, S. (1900). 'The Interpretation of Dreams,' in *The Standard Edition of the Complete Psychological Works*, vols. 4–5. London: The Hogart Press, 1966.
Freud, S. (1905). 'Three Essays on the Theory of Sexuality,' in *The Standard Edition of the Complete Psychological Works*, vol. 7. London: The Hogart Press, 1975.
Freud, S. (1912–1913). 'Totem and Taboo,' in *The Standard Edition of the Complete Psychological Works*, vol. 13. London: The Hogart Press, 1966.
Freud, S. (1914). 'On Narcissism: An Introduction,' in *The Standard Edition of the Complete Psychological Works*, vol. 14. London: The Hogart Press, 1966.
Freud, S. (1920). 'Beyond the Pleasure Principle,' in *The Standard Edition of the Complete Psychological Works*, vol. 18. London: The Hogart Press, 1966.
Freud, S. (1922). '*The Ego and the Id*', in *The Standard Edition of the Complete Psychological Works*, vol. 19. London: The Hogart Press, 1966.
Freud, S. (1927). 'The Future of an Illusion,' in *The Standard Edition of the Complete Psychological Works*, vol. 21. London: The Hogart Press, 1961.
Freud, S. (1928). 'Dostoevsky and Parricide,' in *The Standard Edition of the Complete Psychological Works*, vol. 21. London: The Hogart Press, 1961.
Freud, S. (1929). 'Civilization and its Discontents,' in *The Standard Edition of the Complete Psychological Works*, vol. 21. London: The Hogart Press, 1961.
Fridman, B. D. (1925). '*Osnovnye psichologicheskie vozzreniia Frejda i teoriia istoricheskogo materializma*' (Freud's Main Psychological Views and the Theory of Historical Materialism), in Kornilov, K. N. (ed.). *Psichologiia i marksizm* (Psychology and Marxism). Moscow: Gosizdat (Ital. transl., *Le principali concezioni psicologiche di Freud e la teoria del materialismo storico*, in Angelini, A. (ed.) *Pionieri dell'inconscio in Russia*. Napoli: Liguori, 2002).
Geymonat, L. (1972). *Storia del pensiero filosofico e scientifico*, vol. 11. Milano: Garzanti.
Greenfield, C. C. (1975). 'S. M. Eisenstein's Alexander Nevsky and John Milton's *Paradise Lost*: A Structural Comparison', *Milton Quarterly*, 9 (4), pp. 93–99.
Hautmann, G. (1993). 'Immaginazione e interpretazione', in Di Chiara, G. and Neri, C. (eds.). *Psicoanalisi futura*. Pp. 3–59. Roma: Borla.
Haenen, J., Schrijnemakers, H. and Stufkens, J. (2003). 'Sociocultural Theory and the Practice of Teaching Historical Concepts', in Kozulin, A., Gindis, B., Ageyev, V. S. and Miller, S. M. (eds.). *Vygotsky's Educational Theory in Cultural Context*. Pp. 246–266. Cambridge and New York: Cambridge University Press.

Homskaya, E. D. (2001). *Alexander Romanovich Luria: a Scientific Biography*. New York: Kluwer Academic-Plenum Publisher.

Ionin, L. (1977). 'Pis'mo S.M. Eizenshteina Vyl'gel'mu Raichu', *Sotsiologicheskie issledovaniya*, 1/1977 (1), pp. 181–183 (Ital. transl., W. Reich e S. M. Ejzenštejn. 'Lettere sulla psicoanalisi', *Rassegna Sovietica*, 30 (1), 1979, pp. 3–7.

Iurinets, V. (1925). 'Psychoanalyse und Marxismus', in Sandkühler, Hans Jörg (ed.). *Psychoanalyse und Marxismus: Dokumentation einer Kontroverse*. Frankfurt am Main: Suhrkamp, 1970.

Ivanov, V. V. (1976). *Očerki po istorii semiotiki v SSSR* [*Essays on the History of Semiotics in USSR*). Moscow: Nauka.

Ivanov, V. V. (1977). *Doctor Faust ("Il problema fondamentale" nella teoria dell'arte di S. M. Ejzenštejn)*, in D'Arco, S. A. (ed.). *La cultura nella tradizione russa del XIX e XX secolo*. Pp. 317–358. Torino: Einaudi, 1980.

Jung, C. G. (1908). 'The Content of the Psychoses', in *Collected Works*, vol. 3. Princeton: Princeton University Press, 1960.

Jung, C. G. (1921). 'Psychological Types', in *Collected Works*, vol. 6. Princeton: Princeton University Press, 1971.

Kleiman, N. & Somaini, A. (eds.) (2016), *Sergei M. Eisenstein. Notes for a General History of Cinema*, Amsterdam: Amsterdam University Press.

Köhler, W. (1917). *The Mentality of Apes*. London: Kegan Paul, 1925.

Kollontai, A. (1922). 'Pis'ma k trudiashcheisia molodezhi. Pis'mo vtoroe: Moral' kak orudie klassogo gospodstava i klassovoi bor'by' (Letters to the Working Youth. Second Letter: Morality as a Weapon of Domination and Class Struggle). *Molodaya gvardiia*, 6–7, pp. 128–136.

Kollontai, A. (1923a). 'A proposito del dragone e dell'uccello bianco', in Fracassi, C. (ed.). *Aleksandra Kollontaj e la rivoluzione sessuale*. Roma: Editori Riuniti, 1977.

Kollontai, A. (1923b). 'Largo all'eros alato!', in Fracassi, C. (ed). *Aleksandra Kollontaj e la rivoluzione sessuale*. Roma: Editori Riuniti, 1977.

Koltsova, V. A., Oleinik, Y. N., Gilgen, A. R. and Gilgen, C. K. (eds.) (1996). *Post-Soviet Perspectives on Russian Psychology*. London: Greenwood Press.

Kornilov, K. N. (1922). *Uchenie o reaktsiiach cheloveka* (Reaktologiia) (Theory of Human Reactions [Reactology]). Moscow: Gosizdat.

Kornilov, K. N. (ed.) (1925). *Psikhologiia i marksizm* (Psychology and Marxism). Moscow: Gosizdat.

Kornilov, K. N. (1930). 'Psychology in the Light of Dialectic Materialism', in Murchison, C. (ed.). *Psychologies of 1930*. Worcester, MA: Clark University Press, 1930.

Korsch, K. (1923). *Marxism and Philosophy*. London: NLB, 1970.

Kozulin, A., Gindis, B., Ageyev, V. S. and Miller, S. M. (2003). *Vygotsky's Educational Theory in Cultural Context*. Cambridge, New York: Cambridge University Press.

Kris, E. (1936). 'The Psychology of Caricature'. *International Journal of Psychoanalysis*, 17, pp. 285–303.

Kris, E. (1967). *Ricerche psicoanalitiche sull'arte*. Torino: Einaudi.

Lena Corritore, A. (2021a). 'Sergei Eisenstein's Reading of *Das Traume der Geburt und seine Bedeutung fur die Psychoalalyse* (1924) by Otto Rank', in Ackerman, A. and Aksenjuk, L. (eds.). *Reading with Sergei Eisenstejn*. Montreal: Caboose Books. In press.

Lena Corritore, A. (2021b). 'Sergei Eisenstein's Reading of *Versucht einer Genitaltheorie by Sandor Ferenczi* (1924)', in Ackerman, A. and Aksenjuk, L. (eds.). *Reading with Sergei Eisenstein*. Montreal: Caboose Books. In press.

Lenin, V. I. (1894). *What the "Friends of the People" are and How they Fight the Social-Democrats*, in *Collected Works*, vol. 1. Pp. 129–332. Moscow: Progress Publishers, 1960.

Lenin, V. I. (1909). *Materialism and Empirio-Criticism: Critical Comments on a Reactionary Philosophy*, vol. 14. Moscow: Progress Publishers, 1968.

Leontiev, A. N. (1932). 'The Development of Voluntary Attention in the Child'. *Journal of Genetic Psychology*, 40, pp. 52–81.

Leontiev, A. N. (1965). 'Introduction', in Vygotsky, L. S. (ed.). *The Psychology of Art*. Pp. v–xi. Cambridge, MA: MIT Press, 1971.

Leontiev, A. N. and Luria, A. R. (1956). 'Psikhologicheskie vozzreniya L. S. Vygotskogo' (Psychological Conception of L. S. Vygotsky), in Vygotskii, L. S. (ed.). *Izbrannye psikhologicheskie proizvedeniya*. Pp. 4–36. Moscow: APN RSFSR.

Leontiev, A. N. (1977). *Activity, Consciousness, and Personality*. Englewood Cliffs: Prentice-Hall.

Lévy-Bruhl, L. (1910). *How Natives Think*. New York: Knopf.

Lévy-Bruhl, L. (1922). *Primitive Mentality*. London: Allen & Unwin, 1923.

Lévy-Bruhl, L. (1931). *Primitives and the Supernatural*. New York: Dutton, 1935.

Lewin, K. (1936). *Principles of Topological Psychology*. New York and London: McGraw-Hill.

Lukàcs, G. (1923). *History and Class Consciousness: Studies in Marxist Dialectics*. Cambridge, MA: The MIT press.

Luria, A. R. (1923). 'Psikhoanaliz v svete osnovnykh tendentsiy sovremennoy psikhologii' (Psychoanalysis in the Light of Main Trends of Contemporary Psychology), in Glozman, Zh. M., Leontiev, D. A. and Radkovsky, E. G. (eds.). *Psichologičeskoe nasledie* (*Psychological Legacy*). Pp. 11–29. Moscow: Smysl', 2003.

Luria, A. R. (1925). 'Psychoanalysis as a System of Monistic Psychology', in Luria, A. R. (ed.). *Selected Writings*. Pp. 3–41. White Plains, NY: M. E. Sharpe, 1978.

Luria, A. R. (1932). *The Nature of Human Conflicts, or Emotion, Conflict and Will*. New York: Liveright.

Luria, A. R. (1962). *Higher Cortical Functions in Man*. New York: Basic Books.

Luria, A. R. (1968). *The Mind of a Mnemonist*. New York: Basic Books.

Luria, A. R. (1979). *The Making of Mind: A Personal Account of Soviet Psychology*. Cambridge, MA: Harvard University Press.

Luria, A. R. (1982). *Uno Sguardo sul Passato: Considerazioni Retrospettive sulla Vita di uno Psicologo Sovietico. Firenze: Giunti.*

Luria, E. (1994). *Moy otets A. R. Luria*. Moscow: Gnozis.

Mach, E. (1896). *Contributions to the Analysis of the Sensations*. Chicago, IL: The Open Court.

Manacorda, M. A. (1965). *Il marxismo e l'educazione*, vol. 2. Roma: Armando.

Marti, J. (1976). 'La psychanalyse en Russie et Union Soviètique de 1909 à 1930'. *Critique*, 32 (346), pp. 199–236.

Marx, K. (1844). *Economic and Philosophic Manuscripts of 1844*. New York: International Publishers.

Marx, K. (1867). *Capital: A Critique of Political Economy*, in Marx, K. and Engels, F. (eds.). *Collected Works*, vol I. New York. International Publishers, 1996–1998.

Marx, K. and Engels, F. (1846). *The German Ideology*, in Marx, K. and Engels, F. (eds.). *Collected Works*, vol. 5. New York. International Publishers, 1975.

Mecacci, L. (ed.) (1976). *La psicologia sovietica 1917–1936*. Roma: Editori Riuniti.

Mecacci, L. (1986). 'Introduzione', in Vygotskij, L. S. (ed.). *Lezioni di psicologia*. Roma: Editori Riuniti.

Mecacci, L. (2011). 'Ejzenštejn e Luria'. *Bianco e nero*, (569), pp. 101–105.

Mecacci, L. (2017). *Lev Vygotskij: Sviluppo, educazione e patologia della mente*. Firenze: Giunti.

Metz, C. (1977). *The Imaginary Signifier: Psychoanalysis and the Cinema.* Bloomington: Indiana University Press, Bloomington.
Miller, M. A. (1998). *Freud and the Bolsheviks.* London: Yale University Press.
Montagu, I. (1968). *With Eisenstein in Hollywood.* Berlin, DDR: Seven Seas Books.
Montani, P. (1975). *Dziga Vertov.* Firenze: La Nuova Italia.
Montani, P. (1981). 'Introduzione', in Eisenstein, S. M. *La natura non indifferente*, Montani, P. (ed.). Venezia: Marsilio.
Montani, P. (2016). '"Synthesis" of the Arts or "Friendly Cooperation" between the Arts? The General History of Cinema According to Ejzenštejn', in Kleiman, N. and Somaini, A. (eds.). *Sergei M. Eisentein: Notes for a General History of Cinema.* Pp. 385–391. Amsterdam: Amsterdam University Press.
Münstenberg, H. (1916). *The Photoplay: A Psychological Study.* New York and London: Appleton.
Murchison, C. (ed.) (1930). *Psychologies of 1930.* Worcester, MA: Clark Univ. Press.
Musatti, C. (1963). 'Problemi psicologici del cinema'. *Cinestudio*, (9), pp. 5–7.
Musatti, C. (1969). 'Psicologia degli spettatori al cinema. *Quaderni di Ikon,* n. 7.
Ossicini, A. (1973). 'Intervista', in 'Tutto il mondo è attore'. *Terzoprogramma*, (2/3), pp. 129–135.
Petrovskij, A. V. (1967). 'La critica marxista del freudismo e delle altre correnti soggettivistiche in psicologia', in Mecacci, L. (ed.) (1976). *La psicologia sovietica 1917–1936.* Roma: Editori Riuniti.
Piaget, J. (1923). *The Language and Thought of the Child.* London: Routledge & Kegan Paul, 1979.
Rahmani, L. (1973). *Soviet Psychology: Philosophical, Theoretical, and Experimental Issues.* New York: International Universities Press.
Rank, O. (1912). *The Incest Theme in Literature and Legend: Fundamentals of a Psychology of Literary Creation.* Baltimore, MD: Johns Hopkins University Press, 1991.
Rank, O. (1924). *The Trauma of Birth.* London: Kegan Paul, 1929.
Rank, O. (1932). *Art and Artist: Creative Urge and Personality Development.* New York: Knopf.
Rank, O. and Sachs, H. (1913). *The Significance of Psychoanalysis for the Mental Sciences.* New York: Nervous and Mental Diseases Publ. Co., 1916.
Reich, W. (1927). *The Function of the Orgasm: Sex-Economic Problems of Biological Energy.* New York: Farrar, Straus and Giroux, 1970.
Reich, W. (1929). 'Dialectical Materialism and Psychoanalysis'. *Studies on the Left*, 6, 1966, pp. 736–771.
Reich, W. (1933a). *The Mass Psychology of Fascism.* New York: Farrar, Straus and Giroux, 1970.
Reich, W. (1933b). *Character Analysis.* New York: Simon and Schuster, 1972.
Reich, W. (1936). *The Sexual Revolution: Toward a Self-governing Character Structure.* New York: Farrar, Straus and Giroux, 1945.
Reich, W., Fromm, E. and Sapir, I. (1972). *Psicoanalisi e marxismo.* Roma: Savelli.
Reisner [Rejsner], M. A. (1924). 'Freud e la sua scuola sulla religione', in Rejsner, M. A. *Un giurista sovietico e Freud* (F. Malcovati ed.). Milano: La Salamandra, 1979.
Reisner, M. A. (1925a). 'Sotsial'naya psikhologiia i marksizm' (Social Psychology and Marxism), in Kornilov, K. N. (ed.). *Psikhologiia i marksizm* (Psychology and Marxism). Moscow: Gosizdat.
Reisner [Rejsner], M. A. (1925b). 'La psicologia sociale e la dottrina di Freud, in Rejsner, M. A. *Un giurista sovietico e Freud.* F. Malcovati (ed.). Milano: La Salamandra.

Rice, J. L. (1993). *Freud's Russia: National Identity in the Evolution of Psychoanalysis.* New Brunswick, NJ: Transaction Publishers.
Ruberti, L. (1976). 'Il dibattito su psicoanalisi e marxismo negli anni venti e trenta', *Critica Marxista*, (2), pp. 103–131.
Sachs, H. (1929). 'Zur Psychologie des Films'. *Psychoanalytische Bewegung*, 1 (2), pp. 122–126.
Sapir, I. (1930). 'Freudismo, sociologia e psicologia', in Reich, W., Fromm, E. and Sapir, I. (eds.). *Psicoanalisi e marxismo.* Roma: Savelli, 1972.
Somaini, A. (2011). *Ejzenštejn: Il cinema, le arti, il montaggio.* Torino: Einaudi.
Somaini, A. (2016). Cinema as „Dinamic Mummification" History as Montage: Eisenstein's Media Archaeology, in: Kleiman, N. and Somaini, A. (eds.). *Sergei M. Eisenstein: Notes for a General History of Cinema.* Amsterdam: Amsterdam University Press.
Spielrein, S. (1920). 'Zur Frage der Entstehung und Entwicklung der Lautsprache'. *Zeitschrift für ärztliche Psychoanalyse*, 6, p. 401.
Steila. D. (2007). 'Spinoza e la crisi della psicologia: la riflessione di Lev Vygotskij'. *Intersezioni*, 27 (I), pp. 63–78.
Thalheimer, A. (1926). 'Die Auflösung des Austromarxismus', *Unter dem Banner des Marxismus*, 2 (1–2), pp. 474–557.
Tögel, C. (1989). *Lenin und die Rezeption der Psychoanalyse in der Sovietunion der Zwanziger Jahre* [*Lenin and the reception of psychoanalysis in the Soviet Union in 1920s*]. Retrieved from http://www.freud-biographik.de/frdsu.htm
Trimarchi. G. (2007). *Lev S. Vygotskij: Il "dramma vivente del pensiero" e le premesse della multimedialità.* Milano: Bruno Mondadori.
Trotsky, L. D. (1910). *The Intelligentsia and Socialism.* London: New York Publications.
Trotsky, L. D. (1923). *Rivoluzione e vita quotidiana.* Roma: Samonà e Savelli, 1971.
Trotsky [Trockij], L. D. (1925). *Letteratura e rivoluzione.* Torino: Einaudi.
Tugaybayeva, B. T. (1996). 'Comments on the History of Psychoanalysis in Russia,' in Koltsova, V. A., Oleinik, Y. N., Gilgen, A. R. and Gilgen, C. K. (eds.). *Post-Soviet Perspectives on Russian Psychology.* Pp. 253–266. London: Greenwood Press.
Van Der Veer, R. (2007). 'Vygotsky in Context: 1900–1935', in Daniels, H., Cole, M. and Wertsch, J. (eds.). *The Cambridge Companion to Vygotskij.* Pp. 21–49. New York: Cambridge University Press.
Varjas, A. P. (1925). 'Freidizm i ego kritika s tochki zreniia marksizma' (Freudism and its Criticism from the Point of View of Marxism), in *Dialektika v prirode: Sbornik 1.* Pp.28–62. Vologda: Severnii pechatnik.
Vassilieva, J. (2017). 'Eisenstein and Cultural-Historical Theory', in Neuberger, J. and Somaini, A. (eds.). *The Flying Carpet: Studies on Eisenstein and Russian Cinema in Honor of Naum Kleiman.* Pp. 421–442. Paris: Éditions Mimésis.
Voloshinov, V. N. (1927). *Freudianism: A Marxist Critique.* New York: Academic Press, 1976.
Vygotsky, L. S. (1915). *La Tragedia di Amleto, Principe di Danimarca*, Editori Riuniti, Roma, 1973.
Vygotsky, L. S. (1925a). *The Psychology of Art.* Cambridge, MA: The MIT Press, 1971.
Vygotsky, L. S. (1925b). 'Consciousness as a Problem in the Psychology of Behavior', in *Collected Works*, vol. 3. Pp. 63–79. New York: Plenum Press, 1997.
Vygotsky. L. S. (1926). *Educational Psychology.* Boca Baton, FL: St. Lucie Press, 1997.
Vygotsky. L. S. (1927). 'The Historical Meaning of the Crisis in Psychology: A Methodological Investigation,' in *Collected Works*, vol. 3. Pp. 233–343. New York: Plenum Press, 1997.

Vygotsky, L. S. (1930a). 'The Instrumental Method in Psychology', in *Collected Works*, vol. 3. Pp. 85–90. New York: Plenum Press, 1997.

Vygotsky, L. S. (1930b). 'On Psychological Systems,' in *Collected Works*, vol. 3. Pp. 91–108. New York: Plenum Press, 1997.

Vygotsky, L. S. (1931). 'The History of the Development of Higher Mental Functions,' in *Collected Works*, vol. 4. Pp. 1–251. New York: Plenum Press, 1999.

Vygotsky, L. S (1931–1933). 'The Teaching about Emotions: Historical-Psychological Studies,' in *Collected Works*, vol. 6. Pp. 79–235. New York: Plenum Press, 1999.

Vygotsky, L. S. (1932a). 'On the Problem of the Psychology of the Actor's Creative Work,' in *Collected Works*, vol. 6. Pp. 237–244. New York: Plenum Press, 1999.

Vygotsky [Vygotskij], L. S. (1932b). 'Correnti contemporanee della psicologia', in Mecacci, L. (ed.). *La psicologia sovietica 1917–1936*. Roma: Editori Riuniti, 1976.

Vygotsky, L. S. (1932c). 'Lectures on Psychology,' in *Collected Works*, vol. 1. Pp. 289–358. New York: Plenum Press, 1987.

Vygotsky, L. S. (1934). 'Thinking and Speech,' in *Collected Works*, vol. 1. Pp. 37–285. New York: Plenum Press, 1987.

Vygotsky, L. S. (1935). 'The Problem of Mental Retardation,' in *Collected Works*, vol. 2. Pp. 220–240. New York: Plenum Press, 1993.

Vygotsky, L. S. (1982–1984). *Sobranie sochinenii* (Collected Works), 6 vols. Moscow: Pedagogika.

Vygotsky, L. S. (1987–1999). *Collected Works*. New York: Plenum Press.

Vygotsky, L. S. and Luria, A. R. (1925). 'Introduction' (to the Russian Translation of Freud's *Beyond the Pleasure Principle*), in van der Veer, R. and Valsiner, J. (eds.). *The Vygotsky Reader*. Pp. 10–18. Oxford and Cambridge: Blackwell, 1994.

Vygotsky, L. S. and Luria, A. R. (1930). *Studies on the History of Human Behavior: Ape, Primitive and Child.* Hove: Psychology Press, 2009.

Wertsch, J. V. (1985). *Vygotsky and the Social Formation of Mind*. Cambridge, MA and London: Harvard University Press.

Wilson, A. and Weinstein, L. (1992). 'An Investigation into some Implications of a Vygotskyan Perspective on the Origins of the Mind'. *Journal of the American Psychoanalytic Association,* 40, pp. 349–380, 725–760.

Wilson, A. and Weinstein, L. (1996). 'The Transference and the Zone of Proximal Development.' *Journal of the American Psychoanalytic Association,* 44, pp. 167–200.

Yaroshevsky, M. G. (1996). 'Marxism in Soviet Psychology: The Social Role of Russian Science', in Koltsova, V. A., Oleinik, Y. N., Gilgen, A. R. and Gilgen, C. K. (eds.). *Post-Soviet Perspectives on Russian Psychology*. Pp. 161–186. London: Greenwood Press.

Zalkind, A. B. (1923). 'Vita sessuale e gioventù moderna', in Fracassi, C. (ed.). *Aleksandra Kollontaj e la rivoluzione sessuale*. Roma: Editori Riuniti, 1977.

Zetkin, C. (ed.) (1925). 'My Recollections of Lenin (An interview on the Woman Question)', in *The Emancipation of Women (from the Writings of V. I. Lenin)*. New York: International Publishers, 1966.

Zweig, S. (1931). *Mental Healers: Franz Mesmer, Mary Baker Eddy, Sigmund Freud.* New York: Frederick Ungar, 1962.

Note

1 I am very grateful to Luciano Mecacci for his suggestions and for his friendly support in the realisation of this work.

NAME INDEX

SUBJECT INDEX

For Product Safety Concerns and Information please contact our EU representative GPSR@taylorandfrancis.com
Taylor & Francis Verlag GmbH, Kaufingerstraße 24, 80331 München, Germany

www.ingramcontent.com/pod-product-compliance
Ingram Content Group UK Ltd.
Pitfield, Milton Keynes, MK11 3LW, UK
UKHW020001200926
475702UK00015B/2409
9781032494104